BestMasters

Springer awards „BestMasters" to the best master's theses which have been completed at renowned universities in Germany, Austria, and Switzerland.

The studies received highest marks and were recommended for publication by supervisors. They address current issues from various fields of research in natural sciences, psychology, technology, and economics.

The series addresses practitioners as well as scientists and, in particular, offers guidance for early stage researchers.

Christian Wolf

Audio-Visual Integration in Smooth Pursuit Eye Movements

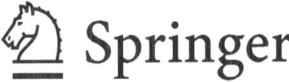 Springer

Christian Wolf
Gießen, Germany

BestMasters
ISBN 978-3-658-08310-6   ISBN 978-3-658-08311-3 (eBook)
DOI 10.1007/978-3-658-08311-3

Library of Congress Control Number: 2014957151

Printed on acid-free paper

Springer is a brand of Springer Fachmedien Wiesbaden
Springer Fachmedien Wiesbaden is part of Springer Science+Business Media
(www.springer.com)

Institutsprofil

Die Psychologie in Giessen kann auf eine lange Tradition verweisen. So wurde 1904 die Deutsche Gesellschaft für Experimentelle Psychologie, aus der später die Deutsche Gesellschaft für Psychologie hervorging, in Giessen gegründet. Von 1911 bis 1927 war Kurt Koffka, Mitbegründer der Gestaltpsychologie, in Giessen tätig. In neuerer Zeit zeichnet sich die Giessener Psychologie als forschungsstark aus, was sich in vielen Rankings widerspiegelt, vor allem auch im Förder-Ranking der Deutschen Forschungsgemeinschaft.

Mit drei Professuren nimmt die Abteilung Allgemeine Psychologie eine zentrale Stellung ein. Die Abteilung um Katja Fiehler, Roland Fleming und Karl Gegenfurtner genießt inzwischen weltweites Renommee durch hervorragende und innovative Arbeit im Bereich der visuellen Wahrnehmung und visuell gesteuerter Handlung. So steht die Abteilung an der Spitze des von der DFG geförderten Sonderforschungsbereichs „Kardinale Mechanismen der Wahrnehmung", eines von der DFG geförderten internationalen Graduiertenkollegs „The brain in action" mit Partnern aus Kanada, und eines von der EU finanzierten Research Training Network zur Wahrnehmung von Oberflächen.

Geleitwort

Die Integration von sensorischen Informationen aus verschiedenen Sinnesmodalitäten ist ein aktuelles und wichtiges Forschungsgebiet in der Psychologie und den Neurowissenschaften. Für die räumliche Lokalisation von Objekten konnte gezeigt werden, dass visuelle und akustische Informationen optimal miteinander kombiniert werden. Dies bedeutet, dass die verschiedenen Informationsquellen umso stärker gewichtet werden, je präziser sie sind und die kombinierte Einschätzung eine höhere Präzision aufweist als die einzelnen Informationsquellen. Da in der Regel visuelle Positionssignale präziser sind als akustische Signale, werden multisensorische Ereignisse eher am Ort der visuellen Position lokalisiert. Dieses Phänomen machen sich z.B. Bauchredner zu Nutze. Verschlechtert man die Präzision der visuellen Information künstlich, werden multisensorische Ereignisse eher am Ort der akustischen Position lokalisiert.

Für die Verarbeitung von Bewegungsinformation und die Steuerung von Augenbewegungen gibt es bislang nur wenige Erkenntnisse darüber, wie und ob visuelle und akustische Informationen integriert werden. Langsame Augenfolgebewegungen dienen dazu, ein bewegtes Objekt mit den Augen zu verfolgen. Bisherige Studien haben gezeigt, dass diese Augenfolge-bewegungen ausschließlich durch visuelle Bewegungssignale gesteuert werden können. Für rein akustische Bewegungssignale war keine Augenfolge-bewegung nachweisbar. In diesen Studien wurden visuelle und akustische Informationen immer getrennt dargeboten, so dass es sein könnte, dass trotzdem visuelle und akustische Signale miteinander integriert werden. Um diese Hypothese zu testen, hat Herr Wolf in seiner Arbeit die Qualität der visuellen Information variiert. Gleichzeitig wurde eine kongruente oder inkongruente akustische Bewegung präsentiert. Wie erwartet, waren die Augenfolgebewegungen umso langsamer je schlechter die Qualität der visuellen Information war. Erstaunlicherweise hatte die akustische Bewegung keinerlei Einfluss auf die Augenbewegungen. Dies bedeutet, dass keine multisensorische Integration von visuellen und akustischen Signalen für die Steuerung von Augenfolgebewegungen stattfindet.

Die Arbeit ist in erster Linie aus der Sicht der Grundlagenforschung von Interesse, zeigt sie doch, dass langsame Augenfolgebewegungen anders verarbeitet werden als die meisten visuelle Reize, indem sie sich einer multisensorischen Bindung sozusagen verweigern. Dies ist insbesondere interessant, weil die multisensorische Integration üblicherweise die Präzision der sensorischen Einschätzung verbessert und bei langsamen Augenfolgebewegungen auf diesen Vorteil verzichtet wird. Die Arbeit hat aber auch wichtige auch praktische Bezüge, etwa bei der ergonomischen Gestaltung von Anzeigen, auf denen bewegte Objekte verfolgt werden müssen (z.B. Flugradar).

PD Dr. Alexander C. Schütz,
Prof. Karl R. Gegenfurtner, Ph.D.

Gießen, Oktober 2014

Table of contents

1. Introduction

1.1. Preface

Anyone who ever started playing a musical instrument has made that experience: At the beginning there is nothing much you can do but lock yourself in a room and practice. Only once you've got accustomed to your instrument and know all its techniques, you can start playing along with others. And maybe, one day, you will find your way into that big orchestra where your own instrument can hardly be detected but where it is of no less importance to the overall emerging music.

The neurosciences are taking a way similar to that of the young musician. While only a few decades ago, our brain has been treated as a multitude of independent modules, it was only recently that scientists began drawing things together and e.g. start to understand how information from different senses are combined into a common percept. This is also reflected in newly established models of human information integration and brain imaging techniques (e.g. multi-voxel pattern analysis) which focus more on the interplay of different neurons, brain areas and senses rather than on their individual activity. Still, we do not yet fully understand the orchestra of neural activity which gives rise to our abilities and our mind.

Indeed, combining different research fields and relating individual abilities is a step towards understanding how the brain works in real world scenarios where nothing is as independent of one another as it is sometimes treated in laboratory settings. For example, imagine the following situation: You're sitting on your desk and pursuing an activity that claims your full concentration, e.g. reading an article or writing a thesis. A fly is disturbing you. It sits down on your monitor and buzzes around your head. In order to catch it (and release it at the window), you need to pursue the fly with your eyes. If you ever tried, you will have realized that pursuing a fly on the flight is a demanding task. Fortunately, you can also hear its buzzing. Does the sound only help you localizing the fly once you lost track? Or does the moving sound directly help you keeping your eyes on the insect?

The present work aims to answer that last question: Does an accompanying sound help us forming a motor command for smooth pursuit eye movements? Therefore, we conducted two experiments on audio-visual integration in smooth pursuit eye movements. The first one tests the influence of the presence and the directional congruency of a moving sound. The second one tests the influence of different visual and auditory velocities.

This work is based on several findings and methods from the smooth pursuit literature, the research field of auditory localization as well as the framework of optimal integration. By drawing these three fields together, we hope to shed light on audio-visual integration in smooth pursuit eye movements.

1.2. Why do we move our eyes?

We move our eyes more often than our heart beats. This is necessary due to the resolution of our retina which depends on the density of photo receptors as well as the convergence from photoreceptors to the consecutive ganglion cells. The distribution of the two photo receptor types - rods and cones - is not uniform across the retina but has its highest density in the fovea, a small region on the retina which exclusively consists of rods. At the same time, most foveal ganglion cells receive input from one rod only, whereas in the periphery the signal from over 100 cones converges to one ganglion cell (Spering & Schmidt, 2012). For these reasons, high visual acuity can only be guaranteed by foveal vision. Peripheral vision on the other hand is rather poor. As a consequence, we need to align our fovea with whatever object interests us in the real world to allow optimal recognition of objects and their properties.

This foveal alignment is achieved by eye movements. Saccades are rapid eye movements that bring objects of interests onto the fovea and thus minimize the difference between visual gaze and target location (position error). They are voluntary as they can be initiated without any specific sensory input. Fixational eye movements help to maintain gaze at a single location. If we start moving our head during fixation, the vestibulo-ocular reflex (VOR) produces an eye movement in the direction opposite to the head in order to maintain gaze and prevent motion blur during self-motion. If, on the other hand, our head remains still and the target starts moving or if we shift our gaze to a target in motion, we would have to move our eye with the same velocity to keep track of it. This is accomplished by smooth pursuit eye movements.

1.3. The pursuit system

1.3.1. Characteristics of smooth pursuit

Smooth pursuit eye movements (pursuit) are slow oculomotor movements which continuously rotate the eye in order to compensate for the retinal slip of the moving target and thus help to keep the tracked target on the fovea and prevent motion blur. Only a few decades ago, it was a common view that pursuit is a mere sensory-motor-reflex which is solely driven by the motion of a target across the retina. Newer studies overcame this view by showing that pursuit is driven by the percept of motion rather than its physical input (Braun, Pracejus, & Gegenfurtner, 2006; Steinbach, 1976). As the fovealization of a moving target has to be initialized out of one's own accord, most authors of recent reviews on eye movement research include smooth pursuit to the voluntary eye movements (Krauzlis, 2004; Schütz, Braun, & Gegenfurtner, 2011), despite the fact that pursuit cannot be elicited in the absence of a target, which indicates that pursuit is not under complete voluntary control (Kowler, 2011). Thus, "pursuit seems to be less voluntary than saccades" (Krauzlis, 2004).

The time between the onset of a target and the execution of an eye movement is called latency. Whereas saccades have a latency of around 150-250ms (Rashbass, 1961), pursuit latencies are somewhat shorter and typically range from 100-200ms. Pursuit latency is influenced by the presence of a distractor moving in another direction (Ferrera & Lisberger, 1995), by target contrast and velocity (Lisberger & Westbrook, 1985; Spering, Kerzel, Braun, Hawken, & Gegenfurtner, 2005) as well as the applied paradigm (Krauzlis & Miles, 1996). In monkeys, latencies are generally shorter for saccades (Paré & Munoz, 1996) as well as for smooth pursuit (Lisberger & Westbrook, 1985).

Smooth pursuit can be divided into two distinct stages. During the first approximately 150ms of the eye movement, the open-loop stage, the eye is accelerated in order to approximate target velocity. During this stage, the eye movement is not yet fully selective for the properties of the moving stimulus, such as its velocity or contrast (Lisberger & Westbrook, 1985; Kowler & McKee, 1987). If two targets start moving in different directions, the initial pursuit response follows the average vector of the two target trajectories (Lisberger & Ferrara, 1997; Gardner & Lisberger, 2001). During the closed-loop phase (also called steady-state), the pursuit response is highly selective due to visual feedback (Lisberger, Morris, & Tychsen, 1987). The pursuit system compares retinal motion (afferent signal) with the motor command that drives the eye (efferent signal or efference copy) and tries to minimize the difference in velocity (retinal slip). Thus, during closed-loop pursuit, eye and target nearly match in their angular velocity and the ratio of eye to target velocity would yield a ratio close to one. This ratio of angular velocities is called the pursuit gain and is a measure for the quality of smooth pursuit.

$$pursuit\ gain = \frac{\vec{\omega}_{eye}}{\vec{\omega}_{target}}$$

Consequently, if pursuit is not perfect (gain < 1), the eye lags behind the target and a positional error is accumulated. To refoveate the target, a catch-up saccade is carried out during the pursuit movement. The positional error, the difference between the target and the current gaze position, is the cue that generally evokes saccades. It has been shown that catch-up saccades are additionally triggered by information about the difference in velocity, the retinal slip. By varying different position and velocity errors, de Brouwer and colleagues could show that our oculomotor system uses both information to compute the time it takes to refoveate the target: the eye crossing time (de Brouwer, Yuksel, Blohm, Missal, & Lefèvre, 2002). For an eye crossing time between 40 and 180ms, the pursuit system is able to account for the compensation on its own and no catch-up saccade is triggered. For values above 180ms, the positional error is relatively high compared to the difference in velocity and the oculomotor systems elicits a saccade to reduce the positional error. For values below 40ms, especially those approaching 0ms,

4

the positional error is minimal but there is still a difference in velocity, i.e. the target is about to overtake the eye and rush ahead. This, as well, can be prevented by a catch-up saccade.

To sum up, especially the pursuit gain can be seen as a quality measurement of smooth pursuit. Pursuit quality (i.e gain) and other pursuit characteristics can be highly influenced by the applied paradigm (section 1.3.2.) as well as the stimulus used (section 1.3.3).

1.3.2. Paradigms to investigate smooth pursuit

One of the key methods to investigate smooth pursuit leads back to Rashbass (1961). He invented the step-ramp paradigm which allows studying pursuit initiation without occurrence of saccades. In the ramp paradigm, a stationary stimulus starts moving in one direction with constant velocity, and a position error is accumulated due to sensory-motor delays. This elicits a catch-up saccade at the beginning of the smooth pursuit trace. In the step-ramp paradigm however, the stimulus is abruptly shifted in one direction before it starts moving in the opposite direction with constant velocity. If target step size and velocity are well coordinated, no catch-up saccade has to be carried out at the beginning of the pursuit trace (Rashbass, 1961). Nowadays, the step-ramp paradigm is the method of choice for investigating pursuit, as it allows studying smooth pursuit initiation without any interference from the saccadic system. Rashbass' main focus however, was not to invent a new paradigm, but to test the independence of pursuit and saccades. He concluded from his research that pursuit responds to the velocity of a target only, whereas saccades are independently stimulated by its position. His work was the basis for the traditional view that saccades and pursuit are complete independent eye movements - a view which dominated the eye movement research for several decades but is nowadays reconsidered due to neural and behavioral similarities (for reviews see Krauzlis, 2004, de Xivry & Lefèvre, 2007).

One of the behavioral similarities between pursuit and saccades is that they are equally influenced by the gap (Krauzlis & Miles, 1996) and overlap paradigm (Erkelens, 2006). In the gap paradigm (Saslow, 1967), the fixation target does not disappear at the same time the saccade target appears, but slightly beforehand. This leads to a decrease in saccadic latency which is dependent on the duration of the gap. There have been observations of express saccades with latencies below 100ms and whose latency distribution is distinct from the latency distribution of normal saccades. Express saccades have been observed in monkeys (Fischer, Boch, & Ramsperger, 1984) as well in humans (Fischer & Rampsberger, 1984). Krauzlis and Miles (1996) combined the gap and step-ramp paradigm to investigate the influence of temporal gaps on smooth pursuit latency. Although no "express pursuit" occurred, pursuit depended on the duration of the gap, similarly as saccades. The counterpart to the gap paradigm is the overlap paradigm where the fixation target is extinguished after the onset of a new target. Erkelens (2006) could show that pursuit and saccade latency highly correlate in the overlap paradigm, but do not in a step paradigm.

1.3.3. The stimulus dependency of smooth pursuit eye movements.

The classical stimulus applied in smooth pursuit research is a small foveal target (for a review see: Lisberger, Morris, & Tychsen, 1987). These targets continuously provide the oculomotor system with information about its position and velocity. As the position error is the signal to drive saccades, pursuit can be interleaved with saccades (Rashbass, 1961) and its decisions can even be overwritten by the saccadic system (Spering, Montagnini, & Gegenfurtner, 2008). To isolate smooth pursuit, you can either apply the step-ramp paradigm (see section 1.3.2) or use a random-dot kinematogram (RDK) as stimulus.

RDKs typically contain several dots that move within a circular aperture. Important parameters are the aperture and dot size, the dot density and lifetime (duration), the noise types (Schütz, Braun, Movshon, & Gegenfurtner, 2010), as well as the coherence of dot velocities and directions. Coherence is usually measured as the percentage of dots which move in the same direction. RDKs have several advantages over other stimuli for smooth pursuit: First, they are not as spatially distinct as foveal targets and thus provide the oculomotor system with no concrete positional information but rather pure information about motion. This is reflected by fewer catch-up saccades during pursuit (Heinen & Watamaniuk, 1998), especially when dot lifetimes are too

6

short for position information to be extracted. Second, they can vary the motion signal by varying velocities (signal itself) as well as coherence (signal-to-noise ratio) and, third, display signal and noise at the same spatial region.

Heinen and Watamaniuk (1998) investigated summation of motion information across the visual field for pursuit using RDKs. They built their research on observations that velocity discrimination is increased when multiple moving targets are present (Verghese & Stone, 1995). Moreover, smooth pursuit acceleration is impaired when pursuing an object relative to a stationary textured background (Keller & Khan, 1986). Kimmig, Miles and Schwarz (1992) could show that this slower acceleration is not due to reduced physical saliency of the target. Another explanation is that the pursuit system averages the motion signal across a larger spatial region and the texture elements of the background provide a zero motion signal. If the motion signal of a larger spatial region is integrated for smooth pursuit, then pursuit should be influenced by the RDK size as well as its dot density. Heinen and Watamaniuk (1998) systematically varied these two parameters. For increasing aperture size, they found increasing eye accelerations as well as decreasing latencies. Additionally, they compared RDK responses to small foveal targets and found consistently higher gains at the end of the open-loop phase with RDKs. In a consecutive study (Watamaniuk & Heinen, 1999), each dot was assigned to one direction from a uniform distribution with the standard deviation of the distribution being an indicator of directional noise. The results show that pursuit follows the average direction within a RDK and eye velocity is lower in high noise (i.e. low coherence) conditions. The authors conclude that the pursuit system integrates across the present motion and follows the vector average in terms of direction and velocity. Others still argue against the usage of RDKs for investigating pursuit as it is difficult to distinguish smooth pursuit from the ocular following response (OFR). OFR appears reflex-like after full field motion with a shorter latency than pursuit and is usually caused by large random dot patterns (Miles, Kawano, & Optican, 1986). However, OFR is not voluntary and can be characterized by its low gain.

Another important stimulus in vision research is the Gabor patch. Gabor patches consist of a sine-wave grating (of luminance or color intensities) covered with a two-dimensional Gaussian. They are of special interest, because they mimic properties of neurons in the visual cortex. Its size is determined by the standard deviation of the Gaussian, its orientation, spatial frequency and phase by the underlying sine-wave. Another important characteristic is its contrast which is defined by the difference between the most and the least luminant part and is thus determined by the amplitude of the sine-wave. Most importantly, it can be changed without affecting the average luminance. That makes Gabor patches optimally suited for contrast experiments.

Based on the finding that humans perceive low contrast stimuli as moving slower (Thompson, 1982; Weiss, Simoncelli, & Adelson 2002) and the high behavioral agreement between motion perception and pursuit (see section 1.3.6), Spering and colleagues (Spering, Kerzel, Braun, Hawken, & Gegenfurtner, 2005) investigated whether low contrast stimuli affect pursuit in a similar way as they do affect perception. They determined individual contrast detection thresholds for identifying the horizontal direction of a moving Gabor patch. In the main experiment, contrast was varied as a multiple of individual detection thresholds. Subjects had to track Gabor patches of different contrasts, spatial frequencies and velocities. Whereas the effect of spatial frequencies on pursuit was rather unsystematic, there was a consistent effect for contrast on pursuit gain, latency and the positional error. With increasing contrast, latency and position error decreased whereas the gain increased as a function of contrast. Additionally, pursuit was interleaved with fewer saccades. The relationship between contrast and gain was as well mediated by target velocity: For slow velocities (1deg/s), gain increases linearly with contrast. For higher velocities (8 and 15deg/s), pursuit gain increases steeply until 2 or 3 times detection threshold and then saturates at higher contrasts. Thus, stimuli contrast can modulate the pursuit response. The authors conclude that for low contrast stimuli, the oculomotor system cannot reliably estimate target velocity. In line with recent models on velocity perception (Weiss, Simoncelli, & Adelson, 2002; see also section 1.3.7), this leads to an underestimation of target speed.

Two targets which have the same luminance are called isoluminant, but humans can usually still tell them apart by their color. Braun and colleagues could show that isoluminant targets cause delayed pursuit onsets and reduced accelerations compared to luminance targets (Braun, Mennie, Schütz, Hawken, & Gegenfurtner, 2008). Thus, pursuit has a preference for targets

8

that are defined by luminance compared to targets that are defined by color. This attribute is also reflected by a study on pursuit target choice by Spering, Montagnini and Gegenfurtner (2008). Subjects had to track a target that was split in a purely luminance-defined and a purely color-defined component. They were told to make an eye movement to the more salient one. Although pursuit decisions were mostly overwritten by saccades which preferred the color-component, the initial pursuit response was biased towards luminance.

1.3.4. Neural pathways of smooth pursuit eye movements

The stimulus dependency of smooth pursuit is informative about its underlying neural mechanisms. Information from different retinal ganglion cells is passed on to the six different layers in the lateral geniculate nucleus (LGN). Magnocellular cells in the first two layers receive input from retinal M-cells. Both type of cells have relatively large receptive fields, they are almost completely insensitive to color but respond to visual motion. Parvocellular and P-cells on the other hand, have small receptive fields and selectively respond to color (Xu, et al., 2001). The smooth pursuit preference for luminance points out that it relies from the magnocellular pathway. However, the facilitated discrimination of isoluminant stimuli during pursuit also argues for a contribution from the parvocellular pathway.

Two important brain regions involved in pursuit are the middle temporal area (MT) as well as medial superior temporal area (MST). MT is located in the superior temporal sulcus and receives input from the magnocellular pathway. It was first described by Dubner and Zeki (1971) who found neurons which selectively responded to direction and to motion in general. Its causal involvement in smooth pursuit was shown by Groh, Born and Newsome (1997). In their study, they stimulated sites in MT and showed that this microstimulation can alter the velocity as well as the direction of smooth pursuit and even evoke pursuit in the absence of a target. Its main task, however, seems to be the initiation of pursuit (open-loop phase) as neurons in MT require retinal motion. If a target is stabilized on the retina during closed-loop pursuit, MT neurons reduce their firing rates, whereas neurons in the dorsal-medial part of MST (MSTd) maintain their firing rate (Newsome, Wurtz,

& Komatsu, 1988) which suggests that it receives extraretinal information, e.g. the efference copy of the eye motor command. Interestingly, receptive fields of neurons in MT are comparatively small compared to neurons in MSTd. Consequently, neurons in MSTd preferentially respond to random dot kinematograms (Komatsu & Wurtz, 1988).

More recent research also emphasized the role of other brain regions for smooth pursuit, among them the frontal pursuit area (FEF$_{SEM}$) and the superior colliculus (SC). FEF$_{SEM}$ is a subregion of the frontal eye fields and receives information from area MST. It seems to be causally involved in pursuit as microstimulation of FEF$_{SEM}$ neurons increase pursuit gain (Tanaka & Lisberger, 2002b). Moreover, its neurons are directionally selective, partly even respond before pursuit onset and their activity is correlated with the behaviorally observed acceleration (Tanaka & Lisberger, 2002). The superior colliculus is a midbrain structure that is supposed to act as a map for orienting movements in general (Carello & Krauzlis, 2004) and particularly for saccades. However, the SC contains neurons in the rostral part which show activity that is related to pursuit (Krauzlis, Basso, & Wurtz, 2000) and it affects smooth pursuit target choice (Nummela & Krauzlis, 2010). FEF and SC, two brain areas that were traditionally associated with saccades. Their contribution to the pursuit pathway, taken together with behavioral similarities between pursuit and saccades argue against two complete distinct eye movement systems.

Most importantly, the pursuit pathway involves area MT and MST which are generally activated when motion is processed, visual as well as auditory motion (section 1.4.2). This is also reflected in the high agreement between smooth pursuit and human motion perception. The relation between the two has only become possible to study since there is a common measure to compare the two: the oculometric function.

1.3.5. Pursuit & psychophysics: The oculometric function

A methodical innovation of great importance for smooth pursuit research was the introduction of the oculometric function by Kowler and McKee (1987). They applied long established methods from psychophysics to eye movement data. Psychophysics has its origin in the 19th century and goes back to the work of

10

Fechner and Weber. It focusses on the relationship between physical stimuli and the sensations and perceptions they cause.

Until the present day, many methods were developed which proved helpful in behavioral research. Typically, psychophysical experiments aim to answer the question whether subjects can detect a stimulus or how good they can distinguish between two stimuli varying in one physical attribute. One of the most applied techniques is the method of constant stimuli where a predefined set of stimuli, which vary slightly in one stimulus property, are randomly and repeatedly presented to the observer. The observer then has to compare the presented stimulus to a standard stimulus and judge which of the two is higher in intensity. Following signal detection theory, the proportion of "more intense" responses can be described as a function of stimulus intensity and can usually be fitted by a cumulative Gaussian. This function is called the psychometric function. Generally, two of the parameters of this cumulative Gaussian are of special interest for psychophysical research: the point of subjective equality (PSE) as well as the slope parameter, the just-noticeable difference (JND).

The PSE is the stimulus intensity which is judged "more intense" in half of the trials, i.e. it is perceived as equivalent to the standard stimulus. The JND on the other hand is a discrimination threshold. It is informative about the slope of the psychometric function. Thus, it reveals how much a stimulus has to deviate from the standard stimulus to be reliably distinguished. Usually the standard deviation of the underlying Gaussian is used for the JND. This allows to directly relate the psychophysical findings to the variability of the sensory percept, which tells how much the sensory signal is corrupted by noise. Moreover, the variability of the sensory percept can also be easily transformed into its reliability – a parameter which is very important in models of multisensory integration (Ernst & Banks, 2002; see also section 1.5.1).

The achievement of Kowler and McKee (1987) was the implementation of the aforementioned psychophysical methods with eye movement data. They applied a velocity discrimination task using the method of constant stimuli. In a separate experiment, they recorded pursuit from the same subjects to the same velocity stimuli. By treating the average pursuit velocity as standard, each pursuit trace could be labelled as faster or slower as the standard response. This results in the dichotomic data that is required to compute a

11

psychometric function based on eye movement data: the oculometric function. This allowed them to study the sensitivity of smooth pursuit, expressed as oculomotor difference threshold. The oculometric function has since been a helpful and frequently used tool in eye movement research, particularly to study the relation between smooth pursuit and motion perception (Spering & Mongtagnini, 2011).

1.3.6. Smooth pursuit and motion perception

The view that performing pursuit requires the presence of physical motion has been questioned by a study of Steinbach (1976). His subjects saw circularly arranged light diodes that started moving as if they belonged to a wheel. Interestingly, when two lights were turned on, subjects perceived a moving wheel and did not pursue the physical spiral trajectory but the perceived center of the wheel. The finding that pursuit agrees with the perceived rather than with the physical stimulus has since been replicated several times. Beutter and Stone (2000) used parallelograms moving behind two rectangular apertures to dissociate between physical and perceived motion. Subjects only saw two lines on each aperture that individually moved up or down, depending on the orientation and direction of the parallelogram. Thus, the physical motion moved in the vertical direction. If the lines are interpreted as a common shape, this would result in a perceived motion that also contains a horizontal component (Adelson & Movshon, 1982). With visible apertures, pursuit followed the perceived direction rather than the physical motion. When the apertures had the same luminance as the background (invisible aperture), no coherent shape could be perceived and pursuit mostly followed the vertical component.

Even stronger evidence comes from an experiment that used the motion after effect to cause smooth pursuit (Braun, Pracejus, & Gegenfurtner, 2006). The motion after effect (MAE) occurs after prolonged exposition to a moving stimulus (adaptation) and describes the afterwards perceived illusory motion of a stationary stimulus in the opposite direction. In the experiment by Braun et al. (2006), subjects had to adopt to a sine-wave grating moving vertically with constant speed of 8.31deg/s. Afterwards they were shown one of the test stimuli which moved at a much lower speed (0.35, 0.69, 1.73deg/s) in one of the vertical directions or which was stationary. Subjects had to pursue each test stimulus and indicate whether it moved up or down. Pursuit traces were then converted into dichotomic up and down responses to compute oculometric functions for the proportion of judgements in the directions of adaptation as a function of test stimulus velocity. Subjects' oculometric functions (PSEs) were consistently shifted towards positive values, i.e. after adaptation subjects needed a stronger motion signal in to elicit pursuit in the direction of adaptation. Most importantly however, were the observed eye movements when showing a stationary stimulus. Here, subjects pursued the illusory motion opposite to adaptation, despite no physical motion was present.

But what is the common nature of pursuit and motion perception? Are they both based on a completely shared sensory signal? If yes, then pursuit and perception should show similar characteristics when comparing the corresponding oculometric and psychometric functions.

This has been tested by Kowler and McKee (1987). By splitting the pursuit trace into 100ms time bins, they could show that the oculomotor difference threshold is not stable but varies over the whole pursuit trace. Whereas it is very high during pursuit initiation (open loop), it decreases continuously until shortly after the mid of the trial (600–700ms), where thus pursuit velocity is best in discriminating between targets of different speed. Moreover, they found that the oculomotor difference threshold in the best time bin is highly consistent with the perceptual difference threshold across different standard velocities. However, they recorded pursuit and perceptual responses in separate sets of trials. Thus, it's not possible to conclude from these results that pursuit and perception both rely on the same sensory signals. It could also be that both rely on different signals that have a comparable amount of noise.

Another consideration predicts that if pursuit and perception share the same neural signal, they would as well share the same noise and consequently the errors of pursuit and perception should be correlated on a trial-by-trial basis. This was tested by two studies that were both published in the same journal at the same time. Despite that, they revealed dissimilar results.

To answer the question whether pursuit and perception are driven by shared neural signals, Stone and Krauzlis (2003) performed a direction discrimination task where a dot moved along the cardinal axes with no or a slight deviation. It was the subjects' task to pursue the dot and afterwards indicate the perceived deviation (clockwise or counterclockwise). Thus, the authors could compare psychometric functions and additionally compute the trial-by-trial agreement between pursuit and saccades. As was shown by Kowler and McKee (1987), the slope parameter for oculometric and psychometric functions were highly similar. Additionally, Stone and Krauzlis (2003) found a high agreement on a trial-by-trial basis. Most important was the statistical difference from chance performance in the absence of any deviation as any agreement in this condition should arise due to shared noise only. Gegenfurtner, Scott, Xing and Hawken (2003) on the other hand didn't find an agreement on a trial-by-trial basis. Their subjects had to pursue small sinusoidal gratings, whose velocity was either increased or decreased for a predefined period, and afterwards indicate whether the stimulus got slower, faster or did not change. Despite a high agreement in the thresholds of pursuit and perception, there was no correlation of errors above 0.1 for any of the five subjects. Thus, these two studies provided contradictory evidence concerning a shared neural signal for pursuit and perception. Still, both studies set up models which consisted of a shared and an independent signal driving pursuit and perception. However, the different finding might also be based on different relationships between pursuit and perception for direction and velocity discrimination.

There is one scenario, however, in which pursuit and perception completely disagree. Both use different computations to take context motion into account. Spering and Gegenfurtner (2007) let subjects track a small Gaussian dot (target) which was surrounded by two vertically oriented sinusoidal gratings (context). At the beginning of each trial, the target moved with the same velocity as the context. After 500ms, the velocity of target and context were independently decreased or increased for 100ms. In addition to pursuing the target, subjects also had to give a perceptual response after each trial whether the target got faster and slower. By this procedure, Spering and Gegenfurtner could investigate how pursuit and perception include context motion in their computation of a velocity signal. Whereas eye movements were only affected by the average of target and contrast motion, perception was mainly affected by its difference. The authors concluded that pursuit and

14

perception differ because they serve different functions: Whereas the perceptual system aims to isolate objects from its background, which can best be achieved by emphasizing velocity differences, the pursuit systems deals with maintaining an optimal fovealization of a target which can best be achieved by averaging across a larger part of the visual field (Spering & Gegenfurtner, 2007).

To sum up, pursuit shows a strong psychophysical consistency with motion perception (Gegenfurtner et al., 2003; Kowler & McKee, 1987; Stone & Krauzlis, 2003) and follows the perceived rather than the physical motion (Beutter & Stone, 2000; Steinbach, 1976). Moreover, illusory motion is sufficient to cause smooth pursuit (Braun et al., 2006). However, they both differ with regard to how different velocities are integrated (Spering & Gegenfurtner, 2007), which might serve as an explanation for the diverging findings on the trial-by-trial correlation as Gegenfurtner et al. (2003) perturbed the target velocity and Stone and Krauzlis (2003) varied the spatial orientation of the target trajectory. The high accordance between pursuit and motion perception is also reflected in computational models which consist of similar components.

1.3.7. Bayesian models of velocity perception and smooth pursuit

Humans often misperceive the velocity of moving objects as to slow if the objects have a low contrast (Thompson, 1982). The same contrast-dependent decrease can be observed in pursuit eye movements (Spering et al., 2005). Weiss, Simoncelli and Adelson (2002) proposed a Bayesian model of visual motion perception that explains these and other perceptual phenomena. Bayesian models are very popular in sensory-motor neuroscience (Vilares & Körding, 2011) as they can easily explain how the brain deals with uncertainty and previous experience and combines both in an optimal motor command. Previous information is expressed in terms of a prior, a distribution of any (mostly) numeric characteristic or object property that describes how likely a certain value is (assumed) to appear in the real-world. The likelihood on the other hand is a distribution which describes the currently available sensory information. Its variance is related to the uncertainty (i.e. inverse of reliability) of the provided sensory signal. Using these two information, the posterior distribution can be computed using Bayesian Inference which takes the reliability of prior and likelihood into account. The maximum or the mean of this posterior distribution is often taken as the estimate of an ideal observer. Thus, this implies that the brain infers information about the physical world from the current sensory signal (likelihood) and previous experience (prior).

The model by Weiss, Simoncelli and Adelson (2002) is based on the assumption that slower velocities are more likely to occur than fast ones (i.e. a prior distribution that is centered on zero) and that there is uncertainty in estimation of velocity from the sensory signal. As the prior is a comparatively broad distribution, any likelihood with few uncertainty would result in a posterior which is located near the likelihood. With increasing uncertainty in the estimation of the sensory signal (broader likelihood), the location of the posterior distribution is shifted towards the prior. Hence, if you have a clear sensory motion signal that is not corrupted by much noise (narrow likelihood), your perceived velocity (posterior) will most likely correspond to the physical one. If, however, the sensory signal is corrupted by noise (e.g. low contrast), there is higher uncertainty in the signal estimation and one will consequently perceive the motion as being slower.

Freeman, Champion and Warren (2010) build up a Bayesian model to explain velocity perception during smooth pursuit. The model differs from other Bayesian models as it considers pursuit target motion as well as relative motion (target relative to background). Moreover, it distinguishes between a measurement and an estimation phase. Their model is able to explain the reduced gain to low-contrast stimuli as well as other eye movement phenomena. Most importantly, the models by Weiss et al. (2002) and Freeman et al. (2010) provide a theoretical basis to study multisensory integration in smooth pursuit eye movements as they make specific predictions about the way different contrast stimuli affect smooth pursuit. This is of special interest as the current framework of multisensory integration (Ernst & Banks, 2002) makes use of these Bayesian statistics and thus might provide insights to the mechanisms that might be involved in a possible multisensory nature of smooth pursuit.

1.4. Auditory localization

To describe the spatial location of any sound source with respect to a listener, three physical parameters are required: azimuth, elevation and distance. Azimuth and elevation give the horizontal and vertical angle of deviation from a listener's line of sight and are fully sufficient to describe the direction of a sound source. The distance gives additional information where along a specific direction a sound source is located. As little is known about auditory distance perception and most studies focus on localizing the direction of a sound source rather than its absolute spatial location, the focus here will be laid on localizing sounds according to azimuth and elevation. A further distinction has to be made between static and dynamic (i.e. moving) sounds.

1.4.1. Auditory localization of static sounds

One of the pioneers of human sound localization was Lord Rayleigh and his work is nowadays often referred to as the *Duplex theory* (1907). He was the first to discover the importance of two binaural difference cues for localization, namely: the Interaural Time (ITD) and Interaural Level Difference (ILD) with the relevance of each cue strongly depending on sound frequency.

Rayleigh reasoned that if a sound source is presented from the side, the head would shadow the sound wave and occlude the path to the far ear, causing a difference in the sound pressure level between the two ears. This cue is called the Interaural Level Difference (ILD). It is most prominent for high pitch tones (Mills, 1960; Macpherson & Middlebrooks, 2002) and increases with sine of the azimuth angle. Thus, the ILD is maximal for an azimuth of ±90deg and frequencies of around 12kHz (Shaw, 1974). The ILD was reported to account for a sound pressure level of up to 35dB (Middlebrooks, Makous, & Green, 1989).

However, for frequencies below 1000Hz, wavelengths are several times larger than the human head which reduces the acoustic shadow and consequently the ILD as Lord Rayleigh was able to compute. Thus, other cues need to be considered to localize low pitch tones. As the speed of sound waves is constant in air, the temporal difference when a sound source reaches each of two ears is informative about the sounds direction. This is referred to as Interaural Time Difference (ITD) or to account for the oscillating characteristic of constant pure tones, as Interaural Phase Difference (IPD). Lord Rayleigh (1907) presented observers with slightly mistuned tuning forks. Physically, this produces a constantly changing phase difference and perceptually results in an auditory motion moving back and forth between the two ears. Assuming the head to be a rigid sphere with the ears as antipodal points, Woodworth (1938) suggested the ITD to be computed as

$$ITD = \frac{r}{c}(\theta + \sin(\theta))$$

where r is the radius, c the speed of sound and θ the azimuth in radians. Although there are more exact mathematical models nowadays which are based on the exact computation of diffraction and consider more than just the shortest way to the far ear (Aaronson & Hartmann, 2014), Woolworth's formula provides sufficiently precise values that correspond well to values measured on a manikin. Only for frequencies below 500Hz, predicted values deviate slightly by a factor of 3/2 (Kuhn, 1977).

In psychoacoustics, a measurement for the precision of sound localization is the Minimum Audible Angle (MAA). The method was first reported by Mills (1958) and later on improved by Hartmann & Rakerd (1989). In a 2AFC task, subjects have to report which of two sound sources (i.e. speakers) is perceived to be on the right or on the left. The angle which can be correctly discriminated in 75% of the trials is called the MAA. Mills (1960) found a bimodal performance in a localization task: MAAs were smallest (about 1deg) for frequencies of 500 and 5000Hz, but increase to 3-4deg for 1500Hz. Mills concludes that this is caused by the fact that ITDs are optimal at low and ILDs optimal at high frequencies - but neither of the cues is good inbetween. Although the duplex theory is defined for pure tones only, Macpherson and Middlebrooks (2002) found a similar pattern for broadband stimuli: For low-pass stimuli, subjects gave high weights for ITDs and low weights for ILDs, a pattern that was reversed for high-pass stimuli. For wideband stimuli, however, ITDs appeared to dominate the localization judgment. Thus, the duplex theory can be used as a framework to auditory localization of pure tones as well as broadband sounds.

Although ITD and ILD provide adequate information for localization tasks in the horizontal dimension (azimuth), their usefulness is limited for judging the vertical dimension (elevation) of a sound source. According to duplex theory, there are numerous possible directions that produce the same ILDs and ITDs, all lying on a cone, the so called "cone of confusion" (Woodworth, 1938). Indeed, several studies have reported front/back confusions (the same angle of azimuth appears to be mirrored relative to the interaural axis) in 6-10% (Makous & Middlebrooks, 1990) or up to 20% (Burger, 1958) of trials. Front/back confusions can be reduced by increasing the sound bandwidth (Butler, 1986). This points out the importance of spectral cues for sound localization, especially in elevation. For azimuth localization, spectral cues are of minor importance (Macpherson & Middlebrooks, 2002).

Spectral cues are monaural cues as they do not require the use of both ears. The sound spectrum is filtered by the head, the torso and especially the outer ear (pinna) and, depending on the direction of the sound source, strengthens or reduces different parts of the frequency spectrum. The function which relates how the ear receives information from any point in space is called head-related transfer function (HRTF). HRTFs can be derived by comparing the recordings from a subject's inner ear with the output of a sound source. Despite the big variability in individual HRTFs, which is most prominent for high frequencies (Wightman & Kistler, 1989a), HRTFs are applied to create 3D sound for video games and other environments. HRTFs recordings are nowadays available for default manikins, e.g. the KEMAR manikin (Gardner & Martin, 1995) or human data in several databases, e.g. the CIPIC database (Algazi, Duda, & Thompson, 2001).

First behavioral evidence that the pinna plays a major role in sound localization was provided by Fisher and Freedman (Fisher & Freedman, 1968). Subjects had to discriminate between eight loudspeakers that were positioned at 45deg angles around them in the horizontal plane. With the head restrained, subjects showed impaired performance when a 10cm tube was inserted in the ear canal and thus prevented any reflections from the pinna. Similar results are reported by Hofmann, Van Riswick and van Opstal (1998). To modify individual HRTFs, subject's pinnae were filled with a synthetic material. Afterwards, their performance was severely impaired for discrimination in elevation but not in azimuth. This impairment was almost completely recovered after wearing the fillings for an adaptation period lasting up to 39 days. This demonstrates the human ability to relearn the spectral cues provided by the pinna. Furthermore, performance was immediately recovered after filling removal, arguing that the old information of spectral cues was not overwritten but complemented by new information.

1.4.2. Auditory localization of dynamic sounds

In contrast to static sounds, any moving sound source not only provides information about its current location but also about its direction and velocity - the attributes to describe physical motion. Whereas the motion sensitivity of the visual system is known for a relatively long time from the motion aftereffect (Sekuler & Pantle, 1967) and electrophysiological recordings in the cat (Hubel & Wiesel, 1962), it still remains a matter of considerable debate whether the human auditory system can process motion at all or whether it simply detects a change in location. The latter view is called the "snapshot theory".

Empirical supports for the snapshot theory are findings from psychoacoustics, where performances in motion discrimination tasks strongly relate to static sound discrimination. Following the method of minimal audible angles (MAA), the equivalent for dynamic stimuli is named the minimal auditory movement angle (MAMA), the minimum change of a moving stimulus that is required for a reliable detection. As do MAAs, MAMAs are lowest for 0deg azimuth and increase with increasing lateralization (Grantham, 1986). MAMAs show the same frequency dependent drop in performance for tonal stimuli around 1300-2000Hz (Perrott & Tucker, 1988). Generally, MAMAs appear to be several times larger than MAAs (Perrott & Musicant, 1977) and performance is significantly downgraded for stimulus presentation shorter than 300ms. Grantham (1986) interpreted this as a minimum integration time required to combine information across multiple static locations. Moreover, MAMAs show a strong U-shaped source velocity dependency, with best values (around 2deg) for velocities between 1 and 10deg/s (Saberi & Perrott, 1990).

Strong evidence for the sensitivity of the human visual system to motion is the motion aftereffect (MAE), the so-called "waterfall illusion". Barlow and

Hill (1963) were the first to show that this phenomenon can be neurophysiologically explained by adaption of direction selective neurons. Although direction selective neurons have not been found for the auditory domain, any behaviorally observed MAE would suggest their existence. Grantham and Wightman (1979) let subjects adapt to auditory motion in the horizontal plane that was simulated via headphones using ITD and ILD. The adaptation stimulus repeatedly appeared 30deg offset to the midline and moved in the opposite direction. Every 10 seconds, this adaptation stimulus was interleaved by a 1 second auditory probe with the same frequency. The probe stimulus was either stationary or moved with 10, 20 or 40deg/s in the same or in the opposite direction. In the low pitch condition (500Hz), subjects reported the stationary probe more often to move in the opposite direction. This wasn't the case for stationary adaptors, ruling out the possibility of a response bias. This effect was more prevalent for higher adaptation velocities and did not exist for high pitch tones (2000Hz). Grantham and Wightman conclude that this is proof for a frequency dependent auditory motion aftereffect (aMAE) that is several times weaker than its visual counterpart but proof for directional selectivity in the auditory system. The aMAE has been also shown to exist for free-field stimuli (Grantham, 1989) and to depend on the spectral and spatial similarity between adaptor and probe stimulus (Dong, Swindale, Zakaruskas, Hayward, & Cynader, 2000). Thus, there is behavioral evidence for the snapshot theory as well as for a motion sensitive auditory system.

This behaviorally found ambiguity propagates to brain imaging studies. At the end of the last century, the first fMRI studies reported auditory motion sensitive brain areas: the right parietal lobe (Griffiths, et al., 1998) as well as the planum temporale (Baumgart, Gaschler-Markefski, Woldorff, Heinze, & Scheich, 1999). Both have been shown to specifically respond to moving sounds. These studies, however, did not rule out the processing of various stationary locations as proposed by the snapshot theory. They compared stationary to moving sounds using a block design. Within each stationary block, the location of the sound did not change. Thus, any difference in activation could be due to the computation of several spatial locations. Smith and colleagues tried to overcome this limitation (Smith, Okada, Saberi, & Hickok, 2004). They simulated moving auditory stimuli by continuously changing the interaural level difference from -12 to 12db (or vice versa). Stationary stimuli were noise bursts with an ILD randomly drawn from a predefined set ranging from -12 to 12db. Stationary and moving stimuli were displayed for 400ms interleaved by 600ms silence. Within each block (8 seconds) in the stationary condition, the fixed ILD values were changing with every stimuli presentation. Thus, the perceived auditory location was varied randomly in discrete steps. They could replicate the activation of the planum temporale and the right parietal lobe for moving stimuli. The stationary stimuli, however, produced an activation that was not distinguishable from the moving sound condition. This result was strengthened by a follow-up study that used an event-related fMRI design combined with neural adaptation (Smith, Saberi, & Hickok, 2007). Hence, these cortex regions seem to be activated by frequently changing spatial locations rather than by auditory motion.

Contrary results were reported by Poirier and colleagues (2005). Like Smith et al. (2004), they simulated motion stimuli by using ILD and contrasted them to static sounds which vary in their spatial locations. For several cortical regions, e.g. planum temporale, the parietal lobes as well as for premotor cortex, they could confirm the increased activation evoked by moving sounds. Most interestingly was an activation in the middle temporal cortex (MT). This region is usually known as the visual motion area as it is specifically activated by visual motion (Dubner & Zeki, 1971). Although this appears to be a strong argument for auditory motion capability, the authors could not rule out that subjects visually imagined the moving sound. Visual imagery is known to activate visual areas similarly but to a lesser extent as real vision. This is also true for the imagination of motion (Goebel, Khorram-Sefat, Muckli, Hacker, & Singer, 1998).

A third possibility which lies between a direction sensitive system and the snapshot theory is that the auditory system is motion sensitive but not direction sensitive. Building up on the observations by Grantham (1992) that motion sensitivity appears to be generally decreased after adaptation, Magezi and colleagues directly compared general motion sensitivity to directional sensitivity using EEG (Magezi, Buetler, Chouiter, Annoni, & Spierer, 2013). They used an adaptation paradigm in which subjects were either adapted to a stationary, rightward, leftward or a bidirectional motion. After each trial, subjects had to judge the direction as well as the intensity of the probe

22

stimulus. At the same time, auditory evoked potentials (AEP) were recorded. Behavioral results could confirm a directional-sensitive aMAE as reported by Grantham and Wightman (1979) as well as decreased motion sensitivity (Grantham, 1992). For the EEG data, AEPs showed no difference between the rightward and the leftward condition. There was, however, a significant difference between the bidirectional and the stationary condition which was correlated with the behaviorally observed decreased motion sensitivity. The authors conclude that our auditory system relies on motion-sensitive, but non-direction selective mechanisms.

Overall, it can be concluded that much is known about the cues and mechanisms involved in static sound localization: interaural difference cues are used to judge the azimuth of a sound whereas spectral cues are informative about the sounds elevation. On the other hand, there is still a considerable amount of debate whether the human auditory system is able to process motion, i.e. whether it just integrates across several locations or whether it is motion but non-direction selective. Here, the auditory motion aftereffect as well as the activation in area MT reveal first insights to auditory motion processing. Interestingly, area MT also processes motion for smooth pursuit. Thus, it should be possible to draw the two together and influence pursuit characteristics by the presence of an auditory stimulus.

1.5. Multisensory Integration

1.5.1. The framework of multisensory integration

One of the most influential models on multisensory integration was proposed by Ernst and Banks (2002). Their model is nowadays often referred to as optimal integration as it suggests that information from different senses are combined in order to minimize uncertainty in the final percept. Assuming independent noise sources with Gaussian variance and uniform Bayesian priors (see section 1.3.7), the weight for the estimate can easily be computed using maximum-likelihood estimation (MLE). An important parameter is the reliability of each sensory cue. It is given by the inverse of the variance. The weight of each sensory estimate, i.e. how much it contributes to the overall percept, is determined by its relative reliability.

Ernst and Banks (2002) tested their model by applying a visual-haptic 2AFC height discrimination task where visual and haptic information are set in conflict. If the psychophysical data is fit to a cumulative Gaussian, then the sensory variance can be retrieved from the discrimination threshold (JND). Its estimate is given by the point of subjective equality (PSE). By testing vision and haptics separately, they could infer estimates and reliabilities haptics and vision under different levels of visual noise. When comparing their model predictions with behavioral data in a condition where visual and haptic information were present, they could show that the observed data follow model predictions.

Since the work of Ernst and Banks (2002), many studies have investigated combination of cues within or across modalities using the framework of optimal integration (Fetsch, Pouget, DeAngilis, & Angelaki, 2012; Helbig & Ernst, 2007; Oruç, Maloney, & Landy, 2003; Reuschel, Drewing, Henriques, Rösler, & Fiehler, 2010). Most of these studies follow the same structure: Two modalities are provided with slightly deviating information. Using psychophysics, one can then measure the resulting percept as well as the estimate, the reliability and the weight of each component.

1.5.2. Audio-visual Integration

One of the most popular phenomena that results from multisensory integration is the ventriloquism effect, the art of making someone's voice appear to come from somewhere else, e.g. a puppet. Alais and Burr (2004) showed that this illusion arises in an audio-visual localization task and can be explained within the framework of optimal integration. Their observers were asked to spatially localize low-contrast Gaussian blobs and sound clicks whose position was simulated using the interaural time difference (ITD). As human vision is usually more precise in localizing as our auditory system, vision appears to dominate sound (visual capture) whenever there is a conflict between the two. However, in situations where the visual information is rather poor, the opposite is true: sound appears to dominate vision.

Whereas the classical ventriloquism effect applies to static locations, Soto-Faraco et al. (Soto-Faraco, Lyons, Gazzaniga, Spence, & Kingstone, 2002) investigated the effect of visual motion on the discrimination of auditory motion directions. Subjects had to indicate the direction of a moving sound source (left or right) accompanied by a simultaneous or slightly delayed visual apparent motion which consisted of two LED flashes. Perceived auditory direction was specifically biased towards visual motion if both motion patterns have been displayed simultaneously. A study by Meyer and Wuerger (2001) analyzed the reversed way: the effect of auditory motion cues on visual motion detection. Subjects were shown RDKs which varied with respect to their motion coherence. At the same time, two lateral speakers were crossfading in volume, simulating the ILD. They could show that visual motion detection was consistently biased towards the auditory direction. Most important, this bias was most eminent for low coherence values. This finding is in line with the models by Weiss et al. (2002) as well as Ernst and Banks (2002). Any low visual coherence value would result in a broad (i.e. unreliable) likelihood and posterior distribution. Consecutively, auditory information should be more emphasized as its relative reliability is comparatively high. On the contrary, if the visual signal is very reliable, the auditory bias on the overall motion percept should be negligible. Meyer and Wuerger (2001) finished their conclusion by stating that "it is conceivable that other visual functions such as the control of eye movements benefit from concurrent auditory & visual motion signals [...]".

1.5.3. Audio-visual motion integration in smooth pursuit eye movements

Up to date, there has been no solid proof of auditory motion integration in smooth pursuit eye movements. A study which investigated audio-visual integration in smooth pursuit comes from Xiao, Wong, Umali and Pomplun (2007). Participants had to track a small blue disc which moved with a constant velocity of 4deg/s on a gray background. Throughout the trial, the target went invisible several times (target blanking) and was either accompanied by a sound with a linearly increasing, a decreasing, a constant pitch or no sound at all. The sound was displayed using speakers that were positioned left and right from the monitor. The authors found higher eye velocities whenever a sound was present with highest eye velocities for the increasing pitch condition. As changes in pitch only appear whenever a sound source changes its distance (i.e. sagittal plane) and tracking took place in the frontal plane, the performance benefit cannot be due to the integration of motion. This effect is most likely based on attentional mechanisms or longer smooth pursuit maintenance. Otherwise a constant sound could not have improved the pursuit gain compared to a no sound condition.

Boucher et al. (Boucher, Lee, Cohen, & Hughes, 2004) recorded ocular tracking responses to a combined LED/speaker device. The device moved by 3deg/s and provided visual information (V), auditory information (A), both (A+V) or no motion stimulus at all (NS). Their results show a clear distinction between trials with visual information present or not. Thus, audio-visual tracking (AV) did not differ from pure visual tracking (V), and auditory tracking (A) did not differ from tracking of an imagined target (NS). This distinction could be found in eye velocity as well as in the number of interleaving saccades. The authors conclude that our auditory system is not equipped with a low-level motion analysis mechanism but might gain access to a high-level motion processing system which might correspond to third-order motion described by Lu and Sperling (1995). However, the work by Boucher et al. (2004) does not consider a variety of important aspects: First, results were based on raw data from 9-16 trials for each subject in each condition. As any effect of auditory motion on pursuit should be comparably tiny, results should be based on a sufficient size of observations. Second, they did neither vary the velocity of the visual nor of the auditory stimulus. As smooth pursuit is very speed dependent, different target velocities should result in estimates which differ from physical velocity, especially for higher values. Third: a reduced gain could be achieved by varying the quality of the signal (e.g. its contrast). Consequently, the applied visual signal was sufficient to produce close to perfect pursuit. Only an oculomotor velocity estimate which is less than the stimulus signal (gain < 1) can yield the possibility for auditory motion to improve smooth pursuit. Moreover, as Alais and Burr (2004) have shown that although vision usually dominates over audition, this pattern can be reversed if the reliability of the visual component is reduced. Taken together, any study which wants to prove an integration of audio-visual motion in pursuit should vary the reliability of the visual signal. Only this could reveal auditory benefits to the overall motion percept (Meyer & Wuerger, 2001).

1.6. Aim of the present study

The present study investigated whether auditory motion signals are integrated with visual information to form a motor command for smooth pursuit. We tested this by combining low contrast visual signals with an accompanying auditory motion signal. We varied the directional (experiment 1) as well as velocity coherence (experiment 2) of both components and analyzed the data using oculometric functions. In line with models of smooth pursuit (Freeman et al., 2010) and experimental observations (Spering et al., 2005), a low contrast signal produced an unreliable visual signal and lower smooth pursuit gains. According to models of multisensory integration (Ernst & Banks, 2002), this was supposed to increase the influence of the auditory component and yield insights whether information from both senses are integrated for smooth pursuit. This would not only reveal further characteristics of the pursuit system, but as pursuit mostly responds to motion, would also help to answer the question whether humans are able to process auditory motion or whether audition processes locations only.

2.   Experiment 1: Audio-visual coherence

Experiment 1 was designed to answer the question whether humans integrate auditory and visual information to form a motor command for smooth pursuit eye movements. If auditory information was integrated and beneficial for the pursuit command, we would expect pursuit to require a lower visual signal for a given gain. This should have been reflected in lower PSE values if both information move coherently (Congruent condition). If the integration was based on the strength of motion rather than its direction, the same effect should have been observed, if both move in opposite directions (Incongruent condition). We included a condition with a stationary sound in order to check for effects of the presence of any auditory signal.

2.1. Methods

2.1.1. Participants

Participants were 8 undergraduate students from Giessen University (mean age = 24, 7 female). Participants gave informed consent and received course credit (5 out of 8) or 8€/h in return. Everyone had normal or corrected to normal vision.

2.1.2. Setup and stimuli

All stimuli have been displayed using the Psychtoolbox (Brainard, 1997; Pelli, 1997) in MATLAB (The Mathworks, Inc., Natick, MA, USA). Visual stimuli were gabor patches with a spatial frequency of sf= 1 cycles/deg and a stimulus size with a Gaussian SD of 0.7deg. Auditory stimuli were pure tones with a frequency of f=1000Hz. They were created and played with MATLAB using the

Psychtoolbox and an HDSPe AIO sound card (RME, Haimhausen, Germany). Sounds were displayed to subjects via Sennheiser HD 280 Pro headphones (Sennheiser electronic GmbH & Co. KG, Wedemark, Germany) and their horizontal location was computed using the interaural time difference (ITD). Auditory motion was simulated by dynamically changing the ITD. Eye movements of the right eye have been recorded with an EyeLink 1000 (SR Research, Osgoode, Ontario, Canada) at a viewing distance of 47cm at 1000Hz.

In session1, contrast values of target Gabor patches varied in five discrete steps from 0.007 to 0.05 Michelson contrast (0.007, 0.01, 0.02, 0.03, and 0.05) and moved with a velocity of 12deg/s. Additionally, there have been distractors moving at 8 or 16deg/s with 0.05 contrast. Gabor patches have been displayed on a neutral gray background with a luminance of 47.6 cd/m². Auditory velocities were adjusted within the experiment by two interleaved staircases for each target contrast and each distractor. Staircase values were updated in the logarithmic domain and had starting values of $10^{0.4}$ and $10^{1.6}$ (approximately 2.5 and 39.8deg/s) and a stepsize of 1.259^2 (about 2.5deg/s). In session2, contrast values and auditory velocities were individually determined from the results of session1 (see section 2.1.5). Contrast values varied logarithmically around the set contrast in seven values from half to twice the contrast.

2.1.3. Data and eye movement analysis

Eye velocity signals were retrieved by differentiating the eye position signal. We used the EyeLink 1000 saccade detection algorithm to determine saccade onset and offset. This algorithm uses a velocity threshold of 22deg/s and an acceleration threshold of 3800deg/s². For pursuit analysis, we removed saccades from velocity traces by linear interpolation. Velocity traces were then filtered by a moving average.

To determine pursuit onset, we fitted a regression line of 80ms to every sample. The best fitting regression line between 10 and 200deg/s² was selected and their interception with the x-axis determined pursuit onset (Schütz, Braun, & Gegenfurtner, 2007). Gain was computed as average velocity from 150ms after the onset (closed-loop) until the end of the trial or until 100ms before the eye reached a horizontal velocity of 0deg/s.

Data from session2 have been converted into dichotomic responses in order to compute oculometric functions. For each subject, we compared the gain of all traces against the median eye trace and converted each trial into a faster or slower response. For oculometric functions, a cumulative Gaussian has been fitted to the data using the psignifit toolbox version 2.5.6 for MATLAB (Wichmann & Hill, 2001a). To compare oculometric functions between the conditions, we applied repeated measures ANOVA whose p-values were corrected according to Greenhouse-Geisser if necessary. All eye movement analysis was executed offline using MATLAB. Inferential statistics were computed in SPSS (Version 21.0).

2.1.4. Procedure

Session1. Each trial consisted of a sequentially displayed visual and auditory stimulus in a randomized order. A fixation cross was displayed at the beginning of each trial to indicate participants that they can initiate a trial by pressing a button on a controller. The visual stimulus was a Gabor patch which appeared on the screen and was stationary for a randomized period of 500 to 1000ms before it started moving horizontally with a constant speed for a randomized duration between 750 and 1250ms (ramp paradigm). The auditory stimulus was a pure tone that was as well first displayed stationary (500-1000ms) and centered (i.e. no ITD) and then started moving for 750-1250ms with a constant velocity. Both stimuli have been separated by the fixation cross that reappeared for 500ms. Subjects were asked to pursue the visual as well as the auditory stimulus and indicate afterwards which of the two moved faster by a response on a keyboard. There have been 350 trials per subject, divided into 4 blocks.

Session2. The second session took place within one week after session1. Session2 was split up into four blocks, one for each condition. Each condition consisted of 180 trials and was defined by the level of audio-visual coherence. Auditory motion either went in the same direction as the Gabor patch (Congruent), in the opposite direction (Incongruent), did not move

(Static) or was not displayed at all (NoSound). The contrast of the Gabor patch as well as the auditory velocity were individually retrieved from session1. Again, a fixation cross indicated participants that they could initiate a trial by pressing a designated button on the controller. The Gabor patch appeared in the screen center, either on its own (NoSound) or simultaneously with a head-centered non-moving sound (Congruent, Incongruent and Static). After a randomized time between 500 and 1000ms, the Gabor patch started moving with a constant velocity (target: 12deg/s, distractor: 8 or 16deg/s) for a randomized time between 750 and 1250ms. Only in the congruent and incongruent condition, the auditory stimulus started moving simultaneously and for the same duration. To ensure that subjects pay attention to the auditory stimulus, they had to report the directional coherence auf audio and visual stimulus after each block.

2.1.5. Parameter estimation

The aim of session1 was to determine individual parameters for Gabor patch contrast as well as the judged auditory velocity. For each subject, we averaged the gain for each contrast and fitted a Weibull function to these values. From this Weibull function, we retrieved the contrast value that corresponds to a gain of 0.7.

For the auditory velocity of each target contrast value, we fitted psychometric functions for the proportion of "auditory motion faster" judgments over different auditory velocities and retrieved PSE and JND values. All auditory velocities were fitted in a log scale. The delogarithmized PSE determines the auditory velocity that is perceived as equally fast as the corresponding Gabor patch. We fitted a weighted linear regression to the 5 (logarithmized) PSE values over the different target contrasts. Residuals of each PSE were weighted by their JNDs. The value of the previously set contrast was entered into the resulting linear equation, which results in the log scaled auditory velocity applied in session2.

To set the auditory velocity for both of the two distractors, we applied the same procedure for the high contrast PSEs (8, 12, 16deg/s). We fitted a weighted regression over the different velocities and extracted the values for 8 and 16deg/s.

2.2 Results

Figure 1 shows an example trial data from session1. Whereas the oculomotor responses to a low contrast visual stimuli varied between low gain pursuit interleaved by saccades and high gain pursuit (Fig 1B), participants could not initiate pursuit with auditory motion only and thus made a sequence of saccades.

Figure 2 shows individual parameters from session1 for the set contrast (Fig 2A) as well as for the judged auditory velocity in log-coordinates (Fig 2B). A table with all individually set parameters can be found in the appendix. Contrary to our expectations, the judged auditory velocity decreases with increasing contrast (Fig 2B). Indeed, 6 out of 8 subjects showed a negative slope. However, the slopes did not significantly differ from zero ($t(7)$ = -1.03, p = .336). We also fitted a weighted linear regression over the different velocities (high contrast) to determine the auditory velocities for the distractors. Here, the judged auditory velocity increased with increasing visual velocity for 7 out of 8 participants. Still, these slopes did not differ from zero either ($t(7)$ = 1.78, p = .118).

The average gain in session2 was 0.71. Data from session2 has been converted into dichotomic oculometric data and fitted to psychometric functions. Example data from one subject (A) and across all subjects (B) is shown in Figure 3. Compared to the NoSound condition, PSEs in the sound conditions cluster around the same value with more PSEs shifted to higher values (Fig 3B). To test the hypothesis that audio-visual integration is beneficial for smooth pursuit, we performed a one-way repeated measures ANOVA on the individual PSEs across participants with the four different conditions as within-subject factor. The ANOVA did not show any significant differences between the conditions, $F(3,21)$ = 1.6, p = .22.

We split up eye traces in time bins of 100ms and computed oculometric functions for each time bin (Fig 4). To test whether any effect of audio-visual

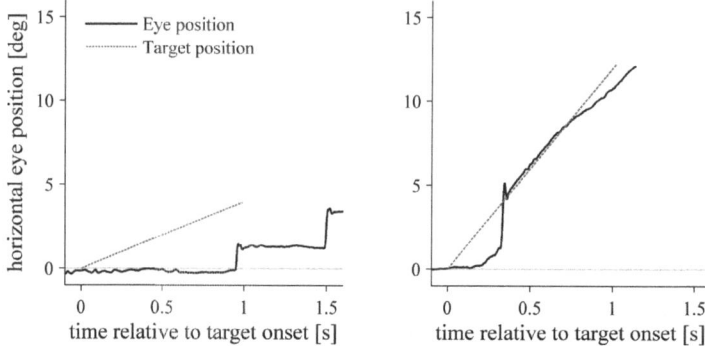

Figure1. Horizontal eye position relative to target onset from an example trial from session1. The solid black line represents the eye position, the dotted gray line the target position. (A): Ocular response to an auditory target moving at 4.7deg/s. Target position is the corresponding coordinate on the screen. (B): Horizontal eye position after onset of a Gabor patch moving with 12deg/s and a Michelson contrast of 0.01

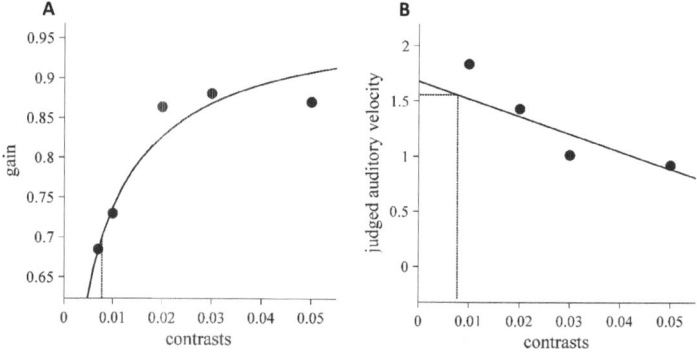

Figure2. Set contrast for session2 (A) and auditory velocity in log scale judged as equally fast for the contrast given in (A). Both data are from subject04. (A): Gain as a function of target Gabor contrast. Data points are arithmetic means for each contrast condition. The solid line represents the fitted Weibull function and the dashed line indicates the contrast which corresponds to a gain of 0.7. (B): Judged auditory velocity as a function of contrast. Data points are PSE values in log coordinates, the solid line represents the weighted linear regression, dashed lines indicate both parameter chosen for session2. One data point is out of the plotted range.

integration might be restricted in time, we performed a two-way repeated measures ANOVA on the PSE values for the within-subject factors condition and time. Only information from 100 to 700ms after pursuit onset was considered, resulting in 6 levels. The results reveal a main effect of time, $F(5,35) = 9.99$, $p = .005$, as well as a significant interaction between the two, $F(15,105) = 2.07$, $p = .017$. The main effect of condition did not yield a significant effect. To pursue the nature of the interaction, we performed post-

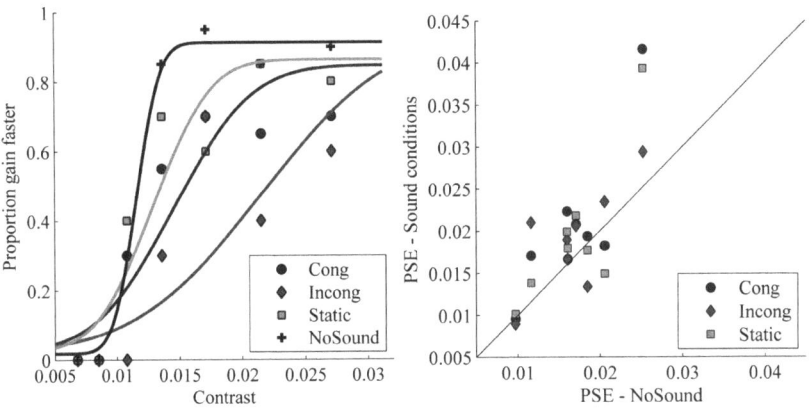

Figure3. Oculometric results for a single (A) and across all participants (B). (A): Data points represent the proportion of eye movement traces faster than the median over different contrast levels for the four different conditions (dark gray: Congruent, medium gray: Incongruent, light gray: Static, black: NoSound). Solid lines represent fitted oculometric functions. Some data points are occluded by data from other conditions. (B): PSEs from the different sound conditions relative to the NoSound condition.

hoc t-tests by comparing the PSEs of the three sound conditions against the NoSound condition in every time bin. We applied a Bonferroni-corrected alpha-level ($\alpha = 0.05/18 = 0.0028$). None of the post-hoc tests revealed a significant result. Still, at pursuit onset, participants tend to be slightly worse in the NoSound condition, whereas they tend to be better in the NoSound condition during the later periods of pursuit (Fig 4).

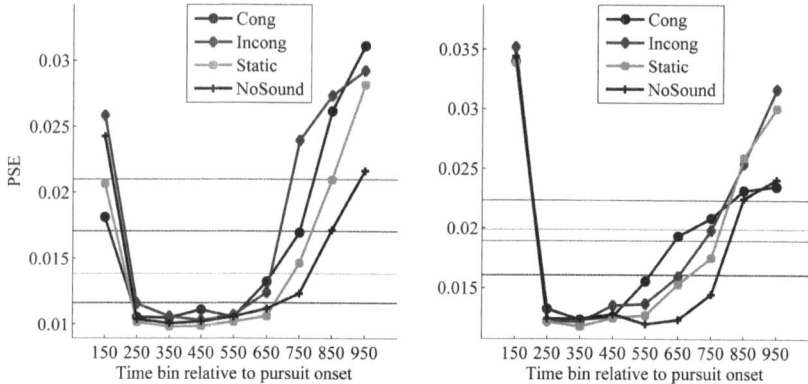

Figure4. PSEs across different time bins [ms] and conditions relative to pursuit onset for two different observers. Time bins have a width of 100ms and are referred by their central position. Data points are PSEs in the respective time bin, dashed lines represent the PSE computed from the complete trace.

2.3. Discussion experiment 1

We investigated whether auditory information is integrated to form an audio-visual smooth pursuit command. We combined an unreliable visual signal with auditory motion signals. Therefore, we first identified for each subject the target contrast which elicited a pursuit gain of 0.7 and the auditory velocity which was perceived as equally fast. Participants were then presented audio-visual signals that had different directional coherences, i.e. compared to the visual target, the auditory motion either moved in the same direction, in the opposite direction, was stationary or was not displayed. We hypothesized to find lower PSE values when visual target and auditory motion move coherently.

We measured the judged auditory velocity for different visual contrasts and different visual velocities. We observed the tendency that perceived velocities increase with increasing stimulus velocity but decrease with increasing contrast. This is contrary to the findings by Thomspon (1982) that the perceived velocity increases with contrast. We cannot rule out the possibility that there is no or a minor effect of the visual contrast on perceived velocity for our stimulus range and that the negative slopes are a result of chance. Another explanation might be that the relationship between perceived velocity and contrast might be fundamentally different during pursuit. The perceived velocity (Thompson, 1982) as well as pursuit gain (Spering et al., 2005) increase with increasing contrast. However, neither Spering and colleagues nor any other study did investigate the contrast-dependent perceived velocity during pursuit. It requires future research to solve this issue.

Overall, we did not find any beneficial effect of an auditory signal on smooth pursuit. This could be due to different reasons: either (I) auditory signals are not integrated for smooth pursuit, (II) our setup is not suitable to test audio-visual integration, (III) participants first have to learn the integration or (IV) any beneficial effect is counteracted by other factors (e.g. the distraction by a sound). The first two points will be discussed in the general discussion (see section 4). The assumption that participants first have to learn the integration seems justified as the audio-visual stimulus is rather artificial. In this case, participants would have to be repeatedly exposed to this kind of audio-visual stimulus. Furthermore, the mere presence of a sound can have an influence on smooth pursuit. Although our experimental conditions were not statistically different from one another, PSE values were mostly lower in the NoSound condition. Moreover, the auditory stimulus was reported to be perceived as unpleasant by two subjects. Thus, the negative effect of a present sound on pursuit could cast an effect that counteracts any audio-visual benefit and is comparatively larger.

To exclude these two possibilities, we performed experiment 2, in which participants were consistently exposed to an audio-visual target which moved in the same direction for three consecutive session taking place on different days. Instead of varying the presence or the directional coherence with the visual target, we varied the velocity of each component.

3. Experiment 2: Audio-visual velocity coherence

In experiment 2, we applied a 2x2-design in which both, the visual and the auditory part of a simultaneous and directionally congruent motion, could independent of one another either be fast or slow. By this, we could compare audio-visual velocity signals which vary in the strength of the auditory as well as the visual motion component. If auditory information is integrated throughout all conditions, we'd expect subjects to require less contrast to perform pursuit. This should be reflected in lower PSE values in the fast auditory conditions (main effect). If, however, integration depends on the coherence of both velocities, we'd expect an interaction in the sense that a pursuit benefit only appears if both components are either fast or slow (interaction). Additionally, we want to test if subjects first have to learn the integration of auditory and visual information. We thus split up the experiment in three consecutive sessions. If integration requires learning, the benefit should become more prominent during the later sessions.

3.1. Methods

3.1.1. Participants

Subjects were nine experienced observers (age: 23years, range: 19-26; 2male) who have previously attended at least one smooth pursuit experiment. None of them has participated in experiment 1. All subjects received 8€/h for participation.

3.1.2. Setup and Stimuli

Setup and Stimuli have been the same as in experiment 1 except that Gabor patch contrast and auditory velocity had fixed values. The (Michelson) contrast of the Gabor patches was set to 0.008, 0.0101, 0.0127, 0.0160, 0.0202, 0.0254 and 0.0320. Gabor patches moved with one of two velocities (12 or 16deg/s). For both visual velocities, we had individually set auditory velocities from experiment 1. For experiment 2, we fixed the auditory velocity to the median judged velocity for the target and the fast distractor (15.8 and 63.1deg/s).

3.1.3. Eye movement analysis & data reduction

Saccade and pursuit detection were the same as in experiment 1. To compute oculometric functions, we normalized traces for the fast and slow visual target independently, as the gain differed significantly between those conditions. Thus, all traces have been dichotomized by comparing each gain with the median of the trials with the same visual target velocity.

For each pursuit trace, we additionally analyzed smooth pursuit characteristics: gain, latency and the number of catch-up saccades during pursuit. To distinguish between pursuit and intersaccadic drifts, which were occasionally detected as pursuit by our algorithm, we defined a pursuit criterion that considers the relation of $gain$ and number of saccades ($nsac$) within each trace:

$$crit_p = gain^2 * (nsac + 1)$$

The distribution of the pursuit criterion $crit_p$ yields a bimodal distribution. The distribution can be found in Figure 5. Values above a critical value of $crit_p \geq 0.2$ were labeled as pursuit. Other trials were not considered for the analysis of pursuit characteristics (e.g. latency, gain, number of catch-up saccades). This applied to 1082 trials (7.2% of total trials). As these trials mostly belonged to the lowest contrast value, there were few if any pursuit observations (5 or less observations for vf-af: 5 out of 9 subjects, vf-as: 7 out of 9, vs-af: 2 out of 9, vs-as: 3 out of 9). Thus, most subjects could not elicit pursuit for the lowest

40

contrast value and we did not include this contrast value for ANOVAs. However, these values were considered for oculometric functions. To compare results from oculometric functions, we applied repeated measures ANOVAs which were corrected according to Greenhouse-Geisser if necessary.

3.1.4. Procedure

A fixation cross indicated to participants that they could initiate a trial by pressing a button on a controller. A Gabor patch appeared on the screen center together with a static sound without any interaural difference. After a randomized time from 500 to 1000ms, both started moving simultaneously and with a constant velocity in the same horizontal direction for a randomized time between 750-1250ms. Gabor patches could either move fast (vf: 16deg/s) or slow (vs: 12deg/s). The same accounts for auditory motion (af: 63.1deg/s; as: 15.8deg/s), resulting in four different conditions (vf-af, vf-as, vs-af and vs-as). Participants had to pursue the target as good as possible. Each observer completed 1740 trials. The experiment was split in three sessions (560 trials) which took place on different days. Each session was split in three blocks with a break after 200 trials. Within each session, the number of trials belonging to the different conditions was balanced and their order randomized.

3.2. Results

3.2.1. Pursuit characteristics

Figure 6 shows the gain as a function of contrast for the four different conditions. Smooth pursuit closed-loop gain increased as a function of visual contrast. Moreover, pursuit gains are higher for the slower visual velocity. We compared the smooth pursuit gain in 6x2x2 repeated measures ANOVA (contrast x visual velocity x auditory velocity). We found a main effect of contrast ($F(5,40) = 45.30$, $p < .001$), a main effect of visual velocity ($F(1,8) = 247.57$, $p < .001$) as well as a significant interaction between visual velocity and the contrast ($F(5,40) = 6.45$, $p = .010$), indicating that pursuit gain

41

increases with target contrast and is higher for (relatively) slower target velocities. However, neither the main effect of auditory velocity, nor any interaction involving the auditory velocity revealed a significant effect.

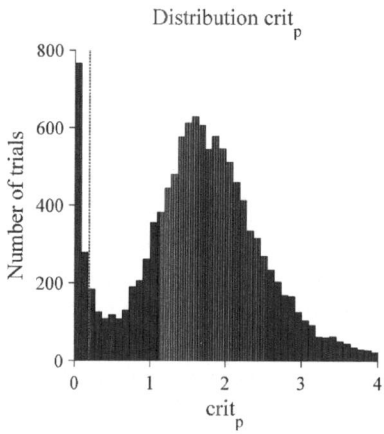

Figure5. Distribution of the pursuit criterion $crit_p$. Values below 0.2 (dotted line) have not been considered for the analysis of pursuit characteristics.

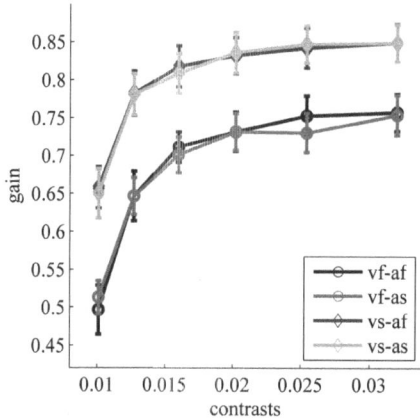

Figure6. Closed-loop smooth pursuit gain as a function of contrast and for different conditions. Data points are between-subject means with one standard error of the mean.

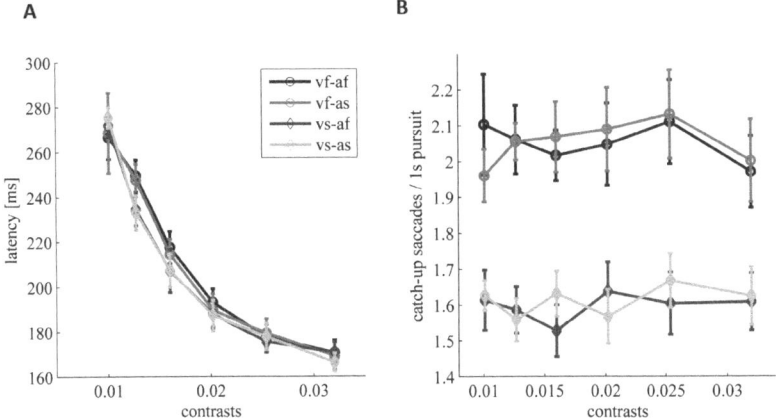

Figure7. Pursuit latency (A) and number of catch-up saccades per second pursuit (B) plotted as a function of contrast. Data points are between-subject means with one standard error.

We applied the same three-way repeated measures ANOVA to the pursuit latency as well as the number of catch-up saccades. For the latency, there was a main effect of contrast only ($F(1,8) = 108.88$, $p < .001$),revealing decreasing latencies with increasing contrast (Fig 7A) whereas for the saccades, we found a main effect of visual velocity ($F(1,8) = 70.73$, $p < .001$). Thus, the number of catch-up saccades seem to depend on the relative target speed only and not on the applied target contrast.

3.2.2. Oculometric results

We computed oculometric functions, one for each participant in each condition. Figure 8 plots individual PSE values for the fast against the slow auditory motion for both visual velocities. Thus, if a strong auditory signal is beneficial for pursuit, we'd expect values to lie underneath the line of origin. Whereas for the slow visual motion, PSE values cluster around the line of origin, values for the fast visual condition are mostly below (7 out of 9). We computed a 2x2 repeated measures ANOVA on the individual

PSE values. We neither found a significant main effect of auditory velocity ($F(1,8) = 1.63$, $p = .238$), nor an interaction ($F(1,8) = 2.87$, $p = .129$), indicating that the auditory signal does not influence smooth pursuit in either way.

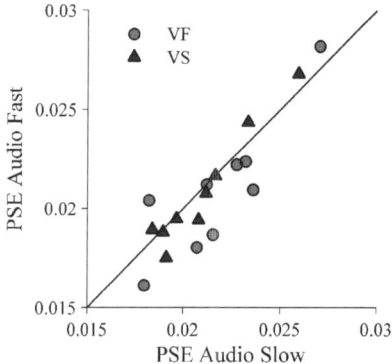

Figure8. Individual PSE values for the fast auditory condition plotted against the slow auditory condition, both, for the slow (triangle) as well as for the fast (circle) visual

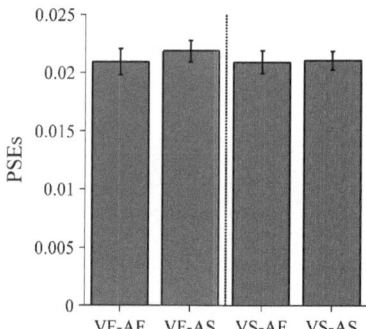

Figure9. Aggregated PSE values for each condition. Bars represent the between-subject average with one standard error. Please note that the difference between the visual conditions is not informative as oculometric functions have been normalized independently (see section 3.1.3.).

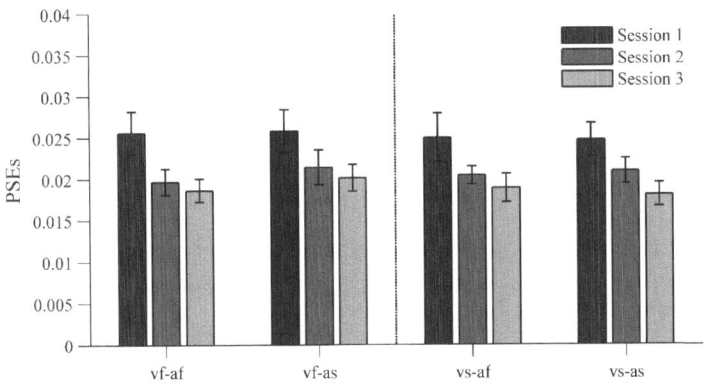

Figure10. Average PSE values for each audio-visual condition split up into different session. Error bars denote one standard error of the mean.

To test the hypothesis that participants require learning the integration of both signals, we split the data into each session and computed oculometric functions for each participant in each of the three sessions. Aggregated data are plotted in figure 10. We performed a three-way repeated measures ANOVA the factors session, visual velocity and auditory velocity. Figure 10 shows a performance benefit over the three sessions. However, the main effect of session does not reach significance ($F(2,16) = 3.08$, $p = .074$). Neither does the auditory main effect ($F(1,8) = 0.98$, $p = .351$), the interaction between session and auditory velocity ($F(2,16) = 0.36$, $p = .701$), or the second order interaction ($F(2,16) = 0.59$, $p = .567$). Thus, although participants slightly improve over the three sessions (not significant), their better performance does not depend on the auditory signals, indicating that participants did not learn the integration of the visual and auditory signal for smooth pursuit.

To test whether any audio-visual effect might be restricted in time, we split the eye trace in time bins of 50ms and computed oculometric functions for every time bin. We performed a three-way repeated measures ANOVA involving 7 different time bins, covering a time from 150-500ms after pursuit onset. Results are plotted in figure 11. The ANOVA revealed a main effect of time ($F(6,48) = 128.59$, $p < .001$), indicating that pursuit performance is

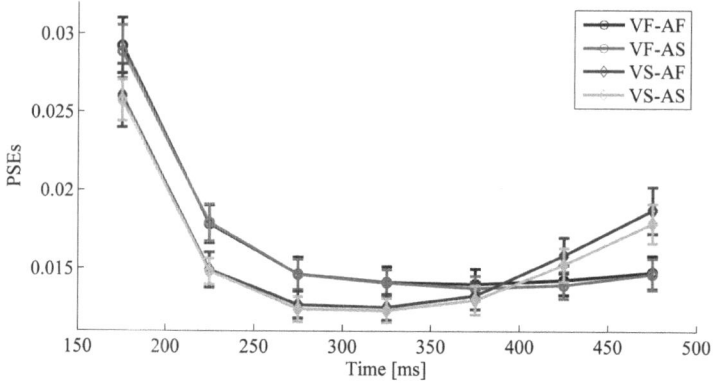

Figure11. PSEs over different time bins for the four different audio-visual conditions. Please note that the difference between the fast and slow visual condition is not informative (see section 3.1.3).

different over time and an interaction between time and visual velocity ($F(6,48)$ = 11.87, p = .002), showing that the time course is different for the two visual velocities. This might lead back to the earlier decrease in performance for the slower visual velocity (Fig 11).

So far, we only tested closed-loop pursuit. To test whether auditory motion signals have an influence on early smooth pursuit, we computed PSE values for open-loop pursuit which were computed from the first 150ms after pursuit onset. On these values, we performed the same two-way repeated measures ANOVA with the two levels of visual and auditory velocity. There was neither any main effect of auditory velocity ($F(1,8)$ = 0.108, p = .75), nor any audio-visual interaction ($F(1,8)$ = 0.25, p = .877). Consequently, for all smooth pursuit parameter, we could not find any auditory or audio-visual effect.

3.3. Discussion experiment 2

We investigated whether audio-visual signals drive pursuit eye movements by independently varying the velocity of the auditory or the visual signal. Any audio-visual integration was assumed to be beneficial for smooth pursuit and be reflected in lower oculometric PSE values. We didn't find any evidence for audio-visual integration, neither an auditory main effect, which would suggest that stronger auditory signals are beneficial to drive the eyes, nor an audio-visual interaction that would be expected when both signals need to match in their velocity in order to be integrated.

Using fixed contrast values additionally allowed us to investigate the contrast dependency of pursuit characteristics and partly replicate the findings by Spering et al. (2005): Gain increased steeply with contrast and saturated at higher values. Latencies were drastically higher for low contrast values and decreased with increasing contrast. Unlike in the experiments from Spering et al. (2005), we found no contrast dependent decrease in the number of catch-up saccades. This is most likely caused by our comparatively narrow range of contrasts whereas Spering et al. (2005) applied contrast values ranging from individual detection threshold up to 100%.

In contrast to the first experiment, we did not apply an adaptive paradigm. Instead, we used fixed values for the contrast as well as for the auditory motion, both derived from adaptive procedures in experiment 1. It is unlikely that our stimuli are responsible for covering any present audio-visual effect. First, subjects in experiment 1 did not have much variance in their set contrast (see table A1, appendix). Second, the contrast values in experiment 2 produced sufficiently large differences in the smooth pursuit gain. Third, most subjects could not initiate pursuit for the lowest contrast value, indicating that detection thresholds were within but at the lower limit of our chosen contrasts. Thus, we applied a visual pursuit signal which was as unreliable as possible.

The auditory velocities were as well retrieved from experiment 1. Although they differed from the physical velocity of our visual stimuli, especially for the fast velocity (visual: 16deg/s, auditory: 63.1deg/s), we could make sure that these velocities perceptually match Gabor patch velocity. Numerical differences probably occurred due the fact that the auditory motion was not explicitly anchored in space. Moreover, minimum audible motion angles (MAMAs) are well above 2deg for velocities around 12 and 16deg/s (Saberi & Perrott, 1990). This would have made auditory velocities of 12 and 16deg/s hard to distinguish. Thus, our stimuli setting were well suited for the purpose of the experiment.

In the discussion of experiment 1 (see section 2.3) we speculated why we didn't find any beneficial effect of audio-visual integration on smooth pursuit. After applying experiment 2, we can now exclude two of the aforementioned possibilities. By splitting up the experiment in three different sessions which were carried out on different days, we wanted to test whether participants need to learn the integration of auditory and visual information. Participants showed a comparatively high increase in performance between the three sessions (figure 10). However, the pattern between the different conditions remained the same within each session, indicating that no learning took place with respect to integration. Any audio-visual learning would have led to an audio-session interaction. We additionally speculated whether any other factors, e.g. the presence of a sound, have an additional effect on pursuit which are bigger and thus overcast any audio-visual integration. The presence of a sound can indeed have high influences on smooth pursuit which seem to be mediated by cognitive aspects (Xiao et al., 2007). To solve this issue, we used an experiment in which auditory and visual motion moved coherently regarding their direction, but only differ with respect to their velocity.

Consequently, we can conclude that humans either do not integrate auditory and visual information for smooth pursuit or our setup is not suitable to study audio-visual integration.

4. General discussion

4.1. Summary of results

Here we tested whether humans integrate auditory and visual signals to form a common audio-visual smooth pursuit motor command. We displayed an unreliable visual component, i.e. low contrast Gabor patches, combined with auditory motion simulated via headphones by varying the interaural time difference (ITD). If audio-visual integration took place, we'd expected pursuit to require a lower visual contras whenever the auditory motion moves in the same direction (experiment 1) or with a faster velocity signal (experiment 2). This should be reflected in lower PSE values in the designated conditions. We haven't found any proof that audio-visual integration occured, neither when varying the directional coherence, nor when varying the velocities of each component. Thus, humans either do not integrate auditory signals for smooth pursuit or they therefore require further information that our setup cannot provide.

4.2. Humans do not integrate for smooth pursuit

The only study who found a beneficial effect of a moving sound on smooth pursuit is the study by Xiao et al. (2007). Their results clearly demonstrate that the presence of even a stationary sound can increase the pursuit gain by about 10%. Although we couldn't replicate this finding, this strongly argues for a higher order mechanism of a sound on smooth pursuit which might be mediated by attention and the sudden onset of a loud sound. Xiao et al. (2007) additionally found higher gains when the visual target was accompanied by a sound with increasing pitch. It is questionable whether their results relate to audio-visual integration. Increasing pitches only occur if an auditory sound source changes its distance relative to an observer. A classic example is the approaching and moving away of an ambulance which results in different pitches depending on the velocity of the ambulance (Doppler Effect). However, for any motion that is restricted to a limited area on the sagittal plane (horizontal motion), changes in distance are neglectable. Thus, any sound source which horizontally moves in front of our eye does hardly lead to changes in pitch. This suggests that their results are based on a higher-order effect but not the mere integration of an auditory and a visual sensory signal. Therefore, no study could ever show audio-visual integration for smooth pursuit and our findings are in line with the literature.

Indeed, one might speculate whether auditory motion can at all be helpful for smooth pursuit. As the research by Heinen and Watamaniuk (1998) as well as Spering and Gegenfurtner (2007) has shown, pursuit averages across a larger part of the retinal field to have a more precise estimate of retinal image motion to reduce retinal slip and foveate the moving target. Whereas the human visual system is very precise in detecting positional offsets or deviations in velocity, our auditory systems is comparably poor and might unsystematically bias any visual estimate. Consequently, our pursuit system might have evolved without considering auditory information.

4.3. Humans do integrate but require positional information

Another possibility is that humans can use auditory signals for smooth pursuit but need additional cues. In our experiments, we only varied the ITD which can give static and dynamic information about azimuth. Stein and Meredith (1993) formulated three principles under which integration of two stimuli from different senses does occur: (i) *the temporal rule*, which states that integration occurs more likely when both stimuli for both senses are displayed at the same time, (ii) *the principle of inverse effectiveness*, which claims that integration is stronger when the unimodal response is comparatively week, and (iii) *the spatial rule*, which states that integration is more likely when both stimuli are displayed at the approximately same location. Whereas both, our visual and auditory stimulus, were displayed at the exact same time and the reliability of the visual signal was low, we thus fulfilled principles (i) and (ii), both stimuli did not arise at the same spatial location.

Our auditory stimulus had a motion component but was not anchored in space, i.e. it did not have a clear spatial location. Therefore, it provided mere information about direction and velocity. Subjects reported perceiving the auditory motion as moving within their head rather than on the screen. There are three possibilities how the setup would need to be changed in order to fulfill the spatial rule formulated by Stein and Meredith (1993). First, headphones could be replaced by speakers located next to the screen whose height is adjusted to fit the horizontal trajectory of the visual target. In this case, the auditory motion would be on the same plane and trajectory as the visual target. Second, both signals could be produced by the same object (e.g. a speaker moving on a rail). Although both signals would spatially and temporally match, it will be difficult to manipulate the visual reliability of the target. Third, when applying a broadband stimulus, a head-related transfer function (HRTF) could be used to manipulate the perceived location of the sound. Here, we used a pure tone with a frequency that is sensitive to changes in ITD. However, when applying broadband stimuli, the reflections of the pinnae can be simulated using HRTFs. As the auditory system is also sensitive to changes in ITD for broadband stimuli (Macpherson & Middlebrooks, 2002), the combination of ITD and HRTF seem an adequate way to control for both, the perceived azimuth and elevation and thus fulfill all the integration principles by Stein and Meredith (1993).

4.4. The multisensory motion circuit

The brain areas which are causally involved in initiating and maintaining pursuit are middle temporal cortex (MT) as well as medial superior temporal area (MST). Interestingly, area MT is also activated when an auditory stimulus is simulated via headphones using the ILD, an interaural cue (Poirier et al., 2005). Our auditory stimulus was comparable to the stimulus by Poirier et al. (2005) as we simulated an interaural cue (ITD) via headphones without any spatial location. Thus, we'd expect that our auditory stimulus lead to an activation in area MT. An increased activation in area MT should produce a stronger smooth pursuit command during pursuit initiation. However, as we didn't find any benefits, neither for open-loop, nor for closed-loop pursuit, we suggest that any possible audio-visual integration for smooth pursuit cannot simply be mediated by a higher activation in MT, but should also include higher order multisensory areas, e.g. the auditory association cortex which was shown to also influence early visual areas (Macaluso, Frith, & Driver, 2000).

4.5. Conclusion

We measured smooth pursuit responses to low contrast targets which were accompanied with auditory motion simulated by using the interaural time delay via headphones. We didn't find any evidence that both signals have been integrated for a multisensory smooth pursuit command. Thus, humans do not integrate visual information with sounds that are defined by direction and velocity only. It requires future research whether integration occurs with auditory motion stimuli which are also localized in space.

5. References

Aaronson, N. L., & Hartmann, W. M. (2014). Testing, correcting, and extending the Woodworth model for interaural time difference. *Journal of the Acoustical Society of America, 135*(2), 817-823.

Adelson, E. H., & Movshon, J. A. (1982). Phenomenal coherence of moving pattern. *Nature, 300*, 523-525.

Alais, D., & Burr, D. (2004). The Vetriloquist Effect Results from Near-Optimal Bimodal Integration. *Current Biology, 14*, 257-262.

Algazi, V. R., Duda, R. O., & Thompson, D. M. (2001). The CIPIC HRTF database. *Proceedings 2001 IEEE Workshop on Applications of Signal Processing to Audio and Electronics* (S. 99-102). New York: New Paltz.

Barlow, H. B., & Hill, R. M. (1963). Evidence for a Physiological Explanation of the Waterfall phenomenon and figural after-effects. *Nature, 200*, 1345-1347.

Baumgart, F., Gaschler-Markefski, B., Woldorff, M. G., Heinze, H. J., & Scheich, H. (1999). A movement-sensitive area in auditory cortey. *Nature, 400*, 724-726.

Berryhill, M. E., Chiu, T., & Hughes, H. C. (2006). Smooth pursuit of nonvisual motion. *Journal of Neurophysiology, 96*, 461-465.

Beutter, B. R., & Stone, L. S. (2000). Motion coherence affects human perception and pursuit similarly. *Visual Neuroscience, 17*, 139-153.

Boucher, L., Lee, A., Cohen, Y. E., & Hughes, H. C. (2004). Ocular tracking as a measure of auditory motion perception. *Journal of Physiology, 98*, 235-248.

Brainard, D. H. (1997). The Psychophysics Toolbox. *Spatial Vision, 10*, 433-436.

Braun, D. I., Mennie, N., Schütz, A. C., Hawken, M. J., & Gegenfurtner, K. R. (2008). Smooth pursuit eye movements to isoluminant targets. *Journal of Neurophysiology, 100*, 1287-1300.

Braun, D. I., Pracejus, L., & Gegenfurtner, K. R. (2006). Motion aftereffect elicits smooth pursuit eye movements. *Journal of Vision, 6*, 671-684.

Burger, J. F. (1958). Front-back discrimination of the hearing system. *Acustica, 8*, 301-302.

Butler, R. A. (1986). The bandwidth effect on monaural and binaural localization. *Hearing Research, 21*, 67-73.

Carello, C. D., & Krauzlis, R. J. (2004). Manipulating intent: Evidence for a causal role of the superior colliculus in target selection. *Neuron, 43*, 575-583.

de Brouwer, S., Yuksel, D., Blohm, G., Missal, M., & Lefèvre, P. (2002). What triggers catch-up saccades during visual tracking? *Journal of Neurophysiology, 87*, 1646-1650.

de Xivry, J. J., & Lefèvre, P. (2007). Saccades and pursuit: two outcomes of a single sensorimotor process. *Journal of Physiology, 584*(1), 11-23.

Dong, C. J., Swindale, N. V., Zakaruskas, P., Hayward, V., & Cynader, M. S. (2000). The auditory motion aftereffect: Its tuning and specificity in the spatial and frequency domains. *Perception & Psychophysics, 62*(5), 1099-1111.

Dubner, R., & Zeki, S. M. (1971). Response properties and receptive fields of cells in an anatomically defined region of the superior temporal sulcus in the monkey. *Brain Research, 35*, 528-532.

Erkelens, C. J. (2006). Coordination of Smooth Pursuit and Saccades. *Vision Research, 46*(1), 163-170.

Ernst, M. O., & Banks, M. S. (2002). Humans integrate visual and haptic information in a statistically optimal fashion. *Nature, 415*, 429-433.

Ferrera, V. P., & Lisberger, S. G. (1995). Attention and target selection for smooth pursuit eye movements. *Journal of Neuroscience, 15*(11), 7472-7484.

Fetsch, C. R., Pouget, A., DeAngelis, G. C., & Angelaki, D. E. (2013). Neural correlates of reliability-based cue weighting during multisensory integration. *Nature Neuroscience, 15*(1), 146-157.

Fischer, B., & Rampsberger, E. (1984). Human express saccades: Extremely short reaction times of goal directed eye movements. *Experimental Brain Research, 57*(1), 191-195.

Fischer, B., Boch, R., & Ramsperger, E. (1984). Express-saccades of the monkey: effect of daily training on probability of occurence and reaction time. *Experimental Brain Research, 55*(2), 232-242.

Fisher, H. G., & Freedman, S. J. (1968). The role of the pinna in auditory localization. *Journal of Auditory Research, 8*, 15-26.

Freeman, T. C., Champion, R. A., & Warren, P. A. (2010). A Bayesian model of perceived head-centered velocity during smooth pursuit eye movement. *Current Biology, 20*, 757-762.

Gardner, J. L., & Lisberger, S. G. (2001). Linked target selection for saccadic and pursuit eye movements. *Journal of Neuroscience, 21*(6), 2075-2084.

Gardner, W. G., & Martin, K. D. (1995). HRTF measurements of a KEMAR. *Journal of the Acoustical Society of America, 97*, 3907-3908.

Gegenfurtner, K. R., Xing, D., Scott, B. H., & Hawken, M. J. (2003). A comparison of pursuit eye movement and perceptual performance in speed discrimination. *Journal of Vision, 3*(11), 865-876.

Goebel, R., Khorram-Sefat, D., Muckli, L., Hacker, H., & Singer, W. (1998). The constructive nature of vision: direct evidence from functional magnetic resonance imaging studies of apparent motion and motion imagery. *European Journal of Neuroscience, 10*, 1563-1573.

Grantham, D. W. (1986). Detection and discrimination of simulated motion of auditory targets in the horizontal plane. *Journal of the Acoustical Society of America, 79*, 1939-1949.

Grantham, D. W. (1989). Motion aftereffects with horizontally moving sound sources in the free field. *Perception and Psychophysics, 45*, 129-136.

Grantham, D. W. (1992). Adaptation of auditory motion in the horizontal plane: effect of prior exposure to motion and motion detectability. *Perception & Psychophysics, 52*, 144-150.

Grantham, D. W., & Wightman, F. L. (1979). Auditory motion aftereffects. *Perception and Psychophysics, 26*, 403-408.

Griffiths, T. D., Rees, G., Rees, A., Green, G. G., Witton, C., Rowe, D., . . . Frackowiak, R. S. (1998). Right parietal corte is involved in the perception of sound movement in humans. *Nature, 1*(1), 74-79.

Groh, J. M., Born, R. T., & Newsome, W. T. (1997). How is a sensory map read out? Effects of microstimulation in visual area MT on saccades and smooth pursuit eye movements. *Journal of Neuroscience, 17*(11), 4312-4330.

Hartmann, W. M., & Rakerd, B. (1989). On the minimum audible angle - A decision theory approach. *Journal of the Acoustical Society of America, 85*(5), 2031-2041.

Heinen, S. J., & Watamaniuk, S. N. (1998). Spatial integration in human smooth pursuit. *Vision Research, 38*, 3785-3794.

Helbig, H. B., & Ernst, M. O. (2007). Optimal integration of shape information from vision and touch. *Experimental Brain Research, 179*, 595-606.

Hofman, P. M., Van Riswick, J. G., & Van Opstal, J. A. (1998). Relearning sound localization with new ears. *Nature, 1*(5), 417-421.

Hubel, D. H., & Wiesel, T. N. (1962). Receptive fields, binocular interaction and functional architecture in the cat's visual cortex. *Journal of Physiology, 160*, 106-154.

Keller, E. L., & Khan, N. S. (1986). Smooth-pursuit initiation in the presence of a textured background in monkey. *Vision Research, 26*(6), 943-955.

Kimmig, H. G., Miles, F. A., & Schwarz, U. (1992). Effects of stationary textured backgrounds on the initiation of pursuit eye movements in monkeys. *Journal of Neurophysiology, 68*(6), 2147-2164.

Komatsu, H., & Wurtz, R. H. (1988). Relation of cortical areas MT and MST to pursuit eye movements. I. Localization and visual properties of neurons. *Journal of Neurophysiology*, 580-603.

Kowler, E. (2011). Eye movements: The past 25 years. *Vision Research, 51*(13), 1457-1483.

Kowler, E., & McKee, S. P. (1987). Sensitivity of smooth eye movements to small differences in target velocity. *Vision Research, 27*(6), 993-1015.

Krauzlis, R. J. (2004). Recasting the smooth pursuit eye movement system. *Journal of Neurophysiology, 91*, 591-603.

Krauzlis, R. J. (2005). The control of voluntary eye movements: New perspectives. *Neuroscientist, 11*(2), 124-137.

Krauzlis, R. J., & Miles, F. A. (1996). Decreases in the latency of smooth pursuit and saccadic eye movements produced by the "gap paradigm" in the monkey. *Vision Research, 13*, 1973-1985.

Krauzlis, R. J., Basso, M. A., & Wurtz, R. H. (2000). Discharge properties of neurons in the rostral superior colliculus of the monkey during smooth-pursuit eye movements. *Journal of Neurophysiology, 84*, 876-891.

Kuhn, G. F. (1977). Physical acoustics and measurements pertaining to directional hearing. *Journal of the Acoustical Society of America, 82*, 157-167.

Lisberger, S. G. (1998). Postsaccadic enhancement of initiation of smooth pursuit eye movements in monkeys. *Journal of Neurophysiology, 79*, 1918-1930.

Lisberger, S. G., & Ferrera, V. P. (1997). Vector averaging for Smooth Pursuit Eye Movements Initiated by Two Moving Targets in Monkeys. *The Journal of Neuroscience, 17*(19), 7490-7502.

Lisberger, S. G., & Westbrook, L. E. (1985). Properties of visual inputs that initiate horizontal smooth pursuit eye movements in monkeys. *Journal of Neuroscience, 5*, 1662-1673.

Lisberger, S. G., Morris, E. J., & Tychsen, L. (1987). Visual motion processing and sensory-motor integration for smooth pursuit eye movements. *Annual Review of Neuroscience, 10*, 97-129.

Lu, Z. L., & Sperling, G. (1995). The functional architecture of human visual motion perception. *Vision Research, 35*, 2697-2722.

Macaluso, E., Frith, C. D., & Driver, J. (2000). Modulation of human visual cortex by crossmodal spatial attention. *Science, 289*, 1206-1208.

Macpherson, E. A., & Middlebrooks, J. C. (2002). Listener weighting of cues for lateral angle: The duplex theory of sound localization revisited. *Journal of the Acoustical Society of America, 111*(5), 2219-2236.

Magezi, D. A., Buetler, K. A., Chouiter, L., Annoni, J. M., & Spierer, L. (2013). electrical neuroimaging during auditory motion aftereffects reveals that auditory motion processing is motion sensitive but not direction selective. *Journal of Neurophysiology, 109*, 321-331.

Makous, J. C., & Middlebrooks, J. C. (1990). Two-dimensional sound localization by human listeners. *Journal of the Acoustical Society of America, 87*(5), 2188-2200.

Meyer, G. F., & Wuerger, S. M. (2001). Cross-modal integration of auditory and visual motion signals. *NeuroReport, 12*(11), 2557-2560.

Middlebrooks, J. C., Makous, J. C., & Green, D. M. (1989). Directional sensitivity of sound-pressure levels in the human ear canal. *Journal of the Acoustical Society of America, 86*, 89-108.

Miles, F. A., Kawano, K., & Optican, L. M. (1986). Short-latency ocular following responses of monkey. I. Dependence on temprospatial properties of visual input. *Journal of Neurophysiology, 56*, 1321-1354.

Mills, A. W. (1958). On the minimum audible angle. *Journal of the Acoustical Society of America, 30*, 237-246.

Mills, A. W. (1960). Lateralization of high frequency tones. *Journal of the Acoustical Society of America, 32*, 132-134.

Newsome, W. T., Wurtz, R. H., & Komatsu, H. (1988). Relation of cortical areas MT and MST to pursuit eye movements. II. Differentiation of retinal from extraretinal inputs. *Journal of Neurophysiology*, 604-620.

Nummela, S. U., & Krauzlis, R. J. (2010). Inactivation of primate superior colliculus biases target choice for smooth pursuit, saccades, and button press responses. *Journal of Neurophysiology, 104*, 1538-1548.

Oruc, I., Maloney, L. T., & Landy, M. S. (2003). Weighted linear cue combination with possibly correlated error. *Vision Research, 43*, 2451-2468.

Paré, M., & Munoz, D. P. (1996). Saccadic Reaction Time in the Monkey. *76*(6), 3666-3681.

Pelli, D. G. (1997). The VideoToolbox software for visual psychophysics: Transforming numbers into movies. *Spatial Vision, 10*, 437-442.

Perrott, D. R., & Musicant, A. D. (1977). Minimum auditory movement angle: binaural localization of moving sound sources. *Journal of the Acoustical Society of America, 62*, 1463-1466.

Perrott, D. R., & Tucker, J. (1988). Minimum audible movement angle as a function of signal frequency and the velocity of the source. *Journal of the Acoustical Society of America, 83*, 1522-1527.

Poirier, C., Collignon, O., DeVolder, A. G., Renier, L., Vanlierde, A., Tranduy, D., & Scheiber, C. (2005). Specific activation of the V5 brain area by auditory motion processing: An fMRI study. *Cognitive Brain Research, 25*, 650-658.

Rashbass, C. (1961). The relationship between saccadic and smooth tracking movements. *Journal of Physiology, 159*, 326-338.

Rayleigh, L. (1907). On our perception of sound direction. *Philosophical Magazine, 13*, 214-232.

Reuschel, J., Drewing, K., Henriques, D. Y., Rösler, F., & Fiehler, K. (2010). Optimal integration of visual and proprioceptive movement information for the perception of trajectory movement. *Experimental Brain Research, 201*, 853-862.

Saberi, K., & Perrott, D. R. (1990). Minimum audible movement angle as a function of sound source trajectory. *Journal of the Acoustical Society of America, 88*(6), 2639-2644.

Saslow, M. G. (1967). Latency for saccadic eye movement. *Journal of Optical Society of America, 57*, 1030-1033.

Schütz, A. C., Braun, D. I., & Gegenfurtner, K. R. (2007). Contrast sensitivity during the initiation of smooth pursuit eye movements. *Vision Research, 47*, 2767-2777.

Schütz, A. C., Braun, D. I., & Gegenfurtner, K. R. (2011). Eye movements and perception: a selective review. *Journal of Vision, 11*(5), 1-30.

Schütz, A. C., Braun, D. I., Movshon, J. A., & Gegenfurtner, K. R. (2010). Does the noise matter? Effects of different kinematogram types on smooth pursuit eye movements and perception. *Journal of Vision, 10*(13), 1-22.

Sekuler, R. W., & Pantle, A. J. (1967). A model for after effects of seen movement. *Vision Research, 88*, 1-11.

Shaw, E. A. (1974). Transformation of sound pressure level from the free field to the eardrum in the horizontal plane. *Journal of the Acoustical Society of America, 56*, 1848-1861.

Smith, K. R., Okada, K., Saberi, K., & Hickok, G. (2004). Human cortical auditory motion areas are not motion selective. *NeuroReport, 15*(9), 1523-1526.

Smith, K. R., Saberi, K., & Hickok, G. (2007). An event-related fMRI study of auditory motion perception: No evidence for a specialized cortical system. *Brain Research, 1150*, 94-99.

Soto-Faraco, S., Lyons, J., Gazzaniga, M., Spence, C., & Kingstone, A. (2002). The ventriloquist in motion; Illusory capture of dynamic information across sensory modalities. *Cognitive Brain Research, 14*, 139-146.

Spering, M., & Gegenfurtner, K. R. (2007). Contrast and assimilation in motion perception and smooth pursuit eye movements. *Journal of Neurophysiology, 98*, 1355-1363.

Spering, M., & Mongtagnini, A. (2011). Do we track what we see? Common versus independent processing for motion perception and smooth pursuit eye movements: a review. *Vision Research, 51*, 836-852.

Spering, M., & Schmidt, T. (2012). *Allgemeine Psychologie 1.* Weinheim: Beltz.

Spering, M., Kerzel, D., Braun, D. I., Hawken, M. J., & Gegenfurtner, K. R. (2005). Effects of contrast on smooth pursuit eye movements. *5*, 455-465.

Spering, M., Montagnini, A., & Gegenfurtner, K. R. (2008). Competition between color and luminance for target selection in smooth pursuit and saccadic eye movements. *Journal of Vision, 8*(15), 1-19.

Stein, B. E., & Meredith, M. A. (1993). *The Merging of the senses.* Cambridge, Massachussets: MIT Press.

Steinbach, M. J. (1976). Pursuing the perceptual rather than the retinal stimulus. *Vision Research, 16*, 1371-1376.

Stone, L. S., & Krauzlis, R. J. (2003). Shared motion signals for human perceptual decisions and acolumotor actions. *Journal of Vision, 3*(11), 725-736.

Tanaka, M., & Lisberger, S. G. (2002). Enhancement of multiple components of pursuit eye movement by microstimulation in the arcuate frontal pursuit area in monkeys. *Journal of Neurophysiology, 87*, 802-818.

Thompson, P. (1982). Perceived rate of movement depends on contrast. *Vision Research, 22*, 377-380.

Verghese, P., & Stone, L. (1995). Combining speed information across space. *Vision Research, 35*, 2811-2823.

Vilares, I., & Körding, K. (2011). Bayesian models: the structure of the world, uncertainty, behavior and the brain. *Annals of the New York Academy of Science, 1224*, 22-39.

Watamaniuk, S. N., & Heinen, S. J. (1999). Human smooth pursuit direction discrimination. *Vision Research, 39*, 59-70.

Weiss, Y., Simoncelli, E. P., & Adelson, E. H. (2002). Motion illusions as optimal percepts. *Nature, 5*(6), 598-604.

Wichmann, F. A., & Hill, N. J. (2001a). The psychometric function: I. Fitting, sampling and goodness-of-fit. *Perception & Psychophysics, 63*(8), 1293-1313.

Wightman, F. L., & Kistler, D. J. (1989a). Headphones simulation of free-field listening. I. Stimulus synthesis. *Journal of the Acoustical Society of America, 85*, 858-867.

Woodworth, R. S. (1938). *Experimental psychology.* New York: Holt.

Xiao, M., Wong, M., Umali, M., & Pomplun, M. (2007). Using eye-tracking to study audio-visual perceptual integration. *Perception, 36*, 1391-1395.

Xu, X., Ichida, J. M., Allison, J. D., Boyd, J. D., Bonds, A. B., & Casagrande, V. A. (2001). A comparison of koniocellular, magnocellular and parvocellular receptive field properties in the lateral geniculate nucleus of the owl monkey. *Journal of Physiology, 531,* 203-218.

6. Appendix

English abstract:

We investigated audio-visual integration in smooth pursuit eye movements. According to established frameworks of multisensory integration, information from different modalities contributes to the common percept according to its reliability. Here, visual reliability was manipulated by reducing the contrast to maximize the influence of the auditory component. We let participants track Gabor patches which were simultaneously displayed with moving sounds simulated via headphones. If auditory information was integrated, we expected pursuit to require less contrast for the same pursuit gain. In two experiments we varied the directional coherence (experiment1) and the velocity of both components (experiment2). Neither did the auditory direction nor did the velocity influence pursuit. We conclude that humans do not integrate auditory motion signals defined by direction and velocity only, but speculate that visual and auditory stimulus therefore have to originate from the same location. (137 words)

German Abstract:

Gemäß etablierten Modellen multisensorischer Integration werden sensorische Informationen einzelner Modalitäten entsprechend ihrer Zuverlässigkeit gewichtet und miteinander integriert. Hier haben wir audio-visuelle Integration bei glatten Augenfolgebewegungen untersucht und die Zuverlässigkeit des visuellen Signals mittels des Kontrastes manipuliert. Versuchspersonen mussten niedrigkontrastige Gaborgitter verfolgen, während zeitgleich ein auditorisches Bewegungssignal via Kopfhörer dargeboten wurde. Sollte Integration stattfinden, hätten wir erwartet, dass die Folgebewegung weniger visuellen Kontrast für eine gleiche Bewegungsstärke benötigt. Dafür haben wir in zwei Experimenten sowohl die Übereinstimmung der Richtung (Experiment1) als auch der Geschwindigkeit beider Komponenten (Experiment2) variiert. In keinem der beiden Experimente zeigte sich ein Einfluss der auditorischen Komponente auf die glatte Augenfolgebewegung. Wir schließen daraus, dass auditorische Bewegung für Folgebewegungen nicht integriert wird, wenn sie ausschließlich über Richtung und Geschwindigkeit definiert ist, aber spekulieren, dass dafür visueller und auditorischer Stimulus von der gleichen räumlichen Position ausgehen müssten.

(138 Wörter)

Table A1. Individually determined contrast and judged auditory velocities from experiment1, session1.

Participant	Set contrast	Judged auditory velocity - target [deg/s]	Judged auditory velocity - slow distractor [deg/s]	Judged auditory velocity - fast distractor [deg/s]
1	0.0164	17.3	15.56	59.16
2	0.0136	19.9	10.61	27.69
3	0.0137	12.3	0.96	17.08
4	0.0078	35.9	6.78	164.66
5	0.0147	13.4	0.00	310241.58
6	0.0173	8.2	3.23	20.60
7	0.0335	10.0	0.92	103.54
8	0.0163	17.8	4.01	71.30

Table A2. Slope parameter from weighted regressions in experiment1 for judged auditory velocities over different contrasts as well as velocities (target and distractor).

$b_{contrast}$	$b_{velocity}$
-11,9853	0,0665
-8,8265	0,0521
22,2316	0,1561
-15,9561	0,1732
-0,1402	1,0916
-90,5949	-0,0723
-5,3163	0,2567
11,2348	0,1023

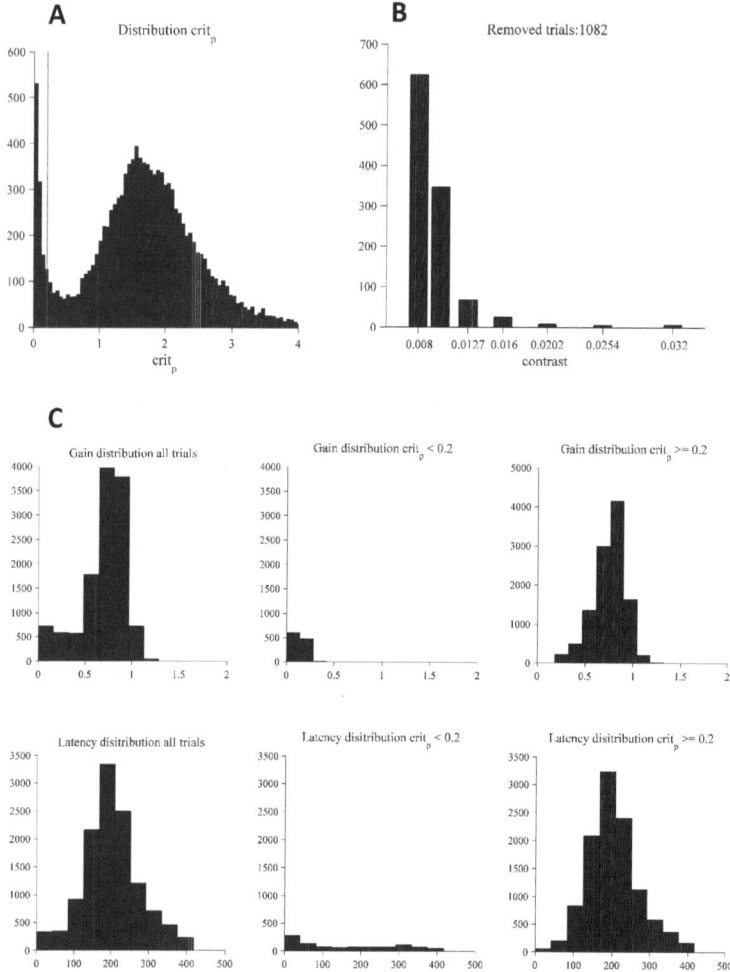

Figure A1. (A) Distribution of the pursuit criterion crit_p. Values below 0.2 (dotted line) have not been considered for the analysis of pursuit characteristics (Figure also shown in figure 5). (B) Number of trials not considered for the analysis of pursuit characteristics split up by contrast. (C) Distribution of gain and latency for all trials (left column), trials not considered for analysis (middle column) and trials considered for analysis (right column).